ENOUGH

A Wild Woman's Tale of Recovery, Discovery, and Transformation.

First published 2025
by Wild Oak Publishing, Somerset, UK.

For permissions requests, please contact
wildoakwellbeing@gmail.com

For my family

"The Bentleys"

Thank you for believing in me, supporting me, and loving me exactly as I am.

Gratitude

I discovered that there are some amazing women out there in the world ready to hold a safe space for me when I was brave enough to ask them to (and sometimes when I couldn't even find the words). Those mentioned here have each gone above and beyond their role as teachers and mentors, often at moments of real vulnerability in my life. They have taught, supported, and guided me with patience, kindness, and humour. A massive thank you to:

Betty Laine (OBE)
Sarah Estelle Turner
Lauren D'Silva

I would also like to mention **Aishling Mooney,** who is a mentor for spiritual entrepreneurs.

She works with angels, humans, and fledgling authors trying to fly for the first time.

Without her belief in me, this book would not have been written.

Finally, I owe an enormous debt of gratitude to **Mother Nature,** especially the trees,

It is with their help that my healing began and continues to this day.

Printed in Dunstable, United Kingdom

64267429R00088

"People who have a strong sense of love and belonging BELIEVE they're WORTHY of love and belonging".

Brene Brown

"If you don't address the wounds of your past, you continue to bleed".

Tina Turner

"I'm not perfect, but I am enough".

Carl Rogers, 1902-1987

Foreword

This is an accidental book. I had only written one chapter for another project, and somehow, it grew legs and started running on its own. It was initially called "Lions and Tigers and Booze, Oh My!" I thought it was a tale about recovery from alcohol dependence with the help of nature and animals. It is still that, but along the way, I discovered it is also a soul journey along a yellow brick road through a scary forest that I conjured for myself. As things evolved, it became clear that the alcohol 'crutch' was just one part of the story and the real essence underneath was WHY I needed to fill the gaping emptiness in my heart, and when I couldn't, why I needed to numb my feelings so much that I could no longer experience happiness and love at all. It led me to the shocking realisation that I believed I just wasn't good enough to be loved.

I felt that I wasn't 'enough.'

I travelled to far-flung places, throwing myself into adventure and looking for answers. It wasn't until I eventually said, "Enough is enough," that I stopped running and started looking within myself. I finally discovered that, actually, I was good enough, holes and all. It took me 40 years to get there. The events and situations in this book are from my perspective and memory, so others may have alternative versions.

This book is for any woman who has ever felt they were not 'enough' in any way, be that not pretty enough, not clever enough, not strong enough, not brave enough, not thin enough, or just not good enough to deserve to be loved completely and unconditionally. It is about finding who you really are under all the different masks you have worn and loving that person in all their naked glory, wobbly bits and all. Loving yourself unconditionally (which is certainly the biggest challenge). Finding the courage to be imperfect and connect with other people because of your vulnerability instead of hiding it. If you have ever needed to fill the emptiness inside with alcohol, drugs, food, sex, exercise, or anything else that has begun to take an unhealthy hold, I understand. For me, each of these 'solutions' eventually led to new problems and an even greater sense of shame, loneliness, and 'un-belonging'. Much of my life was ruled by unbearably intense emotions and the stories I had come to believe about myself and my limitations. On one hand, I didn't feel worthy of love, and on the other, it was impossible to live up to the high expectations I had set for myself. I was bound to fail. A lose-lose situation.

The good news is that I eventually discovered it IS possible to change patterns, habits, and behaviours (and beliefs) and re-route to your best life, the one you really do deserve.

My own journey strayed far from the yellow brick road and meandered down some very dark and rocky paths. Yours will be different (and hopefully, less arduous), but I wish with all my heart that it leads you to the same destination.

Knowing YOU ARE ENOUGH, just as you are.

Contents

ACT 2
AFTER

ACT 3
NOW

Prologue

The heroine of this piece is not a princess but a modern-day woman with all the associated emotions, flaws, strengths, and weaknesses. Sometimes good prevails, and sometimes not. In this real-life tale, I play not only the heroine but sometimes the villain, too. It can feel confusing when we are trying to be the best version of ourselves, but the 'Wicked Witch of the West' lurking inside is determined to get her solo in the spotlight. Please be warned that parts of the story may be a trigger for some people, especially around alcohol, hoarding, and eating issues. Some of the story may cause you to feel disgusted or sad. Me too. But as with all good tales, there is adventure, conflict, and celebration along the way. And humour, which has been my weapon of choice in many battles. Initially, this may seem a somewhat tragic tale, but gradually, it leans more and more towards a comedy.

So, buckle up (it WILL be a bumpy ride), and without further ado, I invite you to join me on this transformational tale.

From self-sabotage to self-love: A story about 'enough-ness'

(Curtain Up)

ACT 1

BEFORE

1

Genie in a Bottle

We all know fairy tales of genies popping out of lamps and granting our wishes. My genie lived in a bottle, and she was certainly no fairy godmother. Her wishes came with a hefty price tag. My story is more gritty Brothers Grimm-style than Hans Christian Anderson (and would definitely not get chosen for a Disney movie plot), but at least I am here on the other side and still able to tell the tale. At this moment in time, it is still in the 'happy ever after' phase, so while the turbulence is at a low, hop up next to me on the magic carpet and let me whizz you back to Southeast London, 13th February 2008.

It is 4 am. I gingerly step out of the taxi with my Bambi-strength legs draped with torn black fishnet tights. I hand over the fare with a blood-stained shaking hand. As I try to get the key into the lock to open my

front door, I realise that my whole body is shaking. In the dark, I wobble my way along the hall to the kitchen, holding onto the walls to support myself. As I open the fridge, the light makes my swollen eyelids sting. I sigh with relief when I see the gloriously chilled bottle is still half full. I quickly pour the liquid into a glass, slopping a fair bit over the rim onto the sticky floor. Clutching the counter to stop my legs from giving way, I take a long gulp. This beautiful nectar has been my ally and crutch for many years, and I really need my friend now. I take another desperate swallow, waiting for the magic to work. I need to numb the pain, the guilt, the shame, and the sadness that is threatening to overwhelm me. Instead, I am hit by a massive wave of nausea and run to the sink to once again empty my agonised stomach. Burning bile and acid pour out of my mouth like liquid poison. "Don't mix these tablets with alcohol," the doctor had firmly said.

I sit there in the darkness, with just one red candle dripping bloody wax onto the wooden table, offering a tiny glimmer of comfort. The thick red velvet curtains are closed, like at the end of a show in a theatre. All finished—time to go home. But I was home and had nowhere else to go. It is the early hours of Valentine's Day. I don't need roses and chocolates and cards; what I need is help. I just don't know how to ask for it. I hear my grandma's broad southern Irish voice echoing from

my childhood: "If you want something done properly, do it yourself". The women in my family prided themselves on being self-sufficient. "Asking for help means you are weak," someone sneers. I don't even know whose voice that is, but it joins the cacophony, chipping away at my brain, all speaking over one another with their chiding voices, each battling to outdo each other; "You're a disgrace, have you no self-control, you should be ashamed of yourself, you're pathetic, no wonder no one loves you" louder and louder until I feel engulfed in noise and negativity. I know I have reached a crossroads. I need to take a mighty sharp turn down another road before it is too late, but maybe it is already too late, as I have pretty much burned all my bridges. I sit at this crossroads, too bone-tired to gather my thoughts and make a decision. I am way past feeling sorry for myself. I don't really feel anything anymore, but gaping emptiness tinged with distant flickerings of shame and despair. Like the flame in front of me, desperately trying to stay alight but slowly running out of oxygen. The truth is, I have failed at life. It is just too hard to get it right. I don't want to die either, though; I just want things to be different. I want a do-over, where I don't muck it all up this time. I want a time-travelling device where I can go back and change things before they all started going pear-shaped.

I still don't know who was listening to me as I finally begged for help in those unforgiving hours between night and day. It was extraordinary. As a long-lapsed Catholic, I no longer had faith that someone was 'watching over me', but somehow, a miracle really did happen, not in a big flash of light or tinkly heavenly voice but quietly and gently. I felt soothed. Held. Comforted. Hopeful.

As dawn winked at me through the curtains. I walked slowly back to the kitchen and poured the rest of the wine down the sink. Never would I have tipped away even the dregs of a wine glass in the past, so watching half a bottle glugging down the plughole was surprising, to say the least. I carefully lined up that bottle alongside the other nine or ten already standing by the door, an empty army of fake confidence that had served their time and done their tours of duty. That was the last glass of wine I ever drank, and now, still sober 17 years later, my whole world has changed. Something or someone decided to give me the helping hand I so needed that fateful morning, and I knew I had a second chance at my life.

I know, it sounds a bit like an overly dramatic plot in a soap opera. So, how did I find myself at that momentous and life-changing moment? How did I get from an intelligent, high-functioning professional woman to a person who had lost all control, both of

themselves and their life? And what's more, did it to herself!

Alcohol was a part of my life from an early age. I remember having a cheeky little Baileys on Christmas Eve that I lapped like a cat and made last two hours (I think I was around 9)—sneaking sips of sherry and glow-in-the-dark yellow 'Snowballs' on Christmas Day. A few Babychams on a camping holiday in Devon with my auntie and uncle, while we sat in our tent playing endless games of 'Careers'. Aged 10 and sharing half a bottle of cherry brandy on holiday in Torremolinos with my new best friend (of three days) when her parents were getting paralytic themselves at the local Bodega (First sip; sweet, fourth sip; vomit-inducing, but keep going, and it gets better again). All of this before I was a teenager, and each time, accompanied by feelings of excitement and bravado. Something grown-up and a bit naughty that miraculously took away all anxiety and flooded my system with happiness. The taste was often revolting, but the heady warmth that came with it and the immediate hit of confidence were already addictive.

To me, alcohol was fun, romantic, and glamorous… anyone around in the 80s who watched Dallas, Dynasty, or even the advert with Joan Collins, Leonard Rossiter, and 'Cinzano' on a plane will know what I mean. Drinking alcohol meant you were sophisticated and in control (how ironic!). It made you laugh and feel

connected with other people. I would often fill a glass with ice and water and walk about the house pretending I was drinking gin, copying Bette Davis or Joan Crawford. Lost in the fantasy of heroines from black and white movies. Leaving smeared rings of sticky strawberry rollerball lip gloss around the rim. Despite living in a rather run-down terraced council house, we had a posh cocktail cabinet filled to the brim with shiny glasses and multi-coloured glittering bottles of liquid magic. It was so easy to drink some and refill with water, hoping no one would notice!

The one drink I have never been able to stomach is whiskey. My mum sometimes used to smell of that, along with the cigarettes. People on film made smoking look cool, but of course, you couldn't smell it. The combination of Teacher's Highland Cream Whisky and Lambert and Butler fags is a vile bouquet that would often preface an ugly scene in my house. It is a scent combination sure to jolt me into a 'fight or flight' reaction (even to this day). The 'freeze' option was no use to me, as that usually meant pain. If I could run, I did. If I couldn't, I sat in a chair and kicked my legs as hard as possible so my mum couldn't get close enough to do much damage. If my grandma were visiting, she would try to intervene, but my mother was filled with such anger towards me that she was not easy to restrain or fight off. I remember seeing a TV advert for

'Childline' with Esther Rantzen and sometimes fantasised about calling it, but the thought of being taken away and put into care was more frightening than managing the violence. Plus, the one phone in the house had a lock on it in case I ran up the bill by chatting to friends. It was the old type of landline handset, where you had to turn the dial and listen to it 'click' its way back round. In my teens, I perfected a very useful technique of lifting the receiver and clicking the little black bits the correct number of times for each number. It was tricky and time-consuming, but I was a very determined young lady, which resulted in many covert conversations with my first love in Alderney (Channel Islands), and no one was ever any the wiser.

I became very adept at reading faces and body language and was highly sensitive to changes in energy and emotions. My mother was unpredictable, and her moods mercurial, so I always had to be on guard, just in case. Sometimes, she would be funny and entertaining, but it was hard to relax and trust this version as, more often than not, there would be a volcanic fury simmering inside her. As I was the only other living creature in the house, I bore the brunt of it. At this stage, my magic "Genie of the bottle" had not properly made herself known as my superhero ally. At this age, I fought my battles alone.

2

Dysfunctional Family Holidays

Family Christmases were usually just my mum, my grandma (Nanny/Helen), and me, but sometimes we joined my auntie and uncle at their house, and they often had visitors. It was a double-edged sword in many ways. I loved being in a house that was clean and uncluttered (unlike my own), and my auntie was a good cook (unlike my mum), so we had proper food cooked from scratch. Invariably, though, there would come a point when everyone had had quite a few alcoholic 'bevvies' and I was instructed to perform and sing for my supper (this would be at my mum's insistence, as I am sure no one else was bothered at all).

My mum had always wanted to be a singer, a dancer, on the stage, in the movies.... You name it, she had

wanted to do it. She had a nice singing voice and had been a good Irish and ballroom dancer, but when she was young, opportunities to be a performer for a living didn't often arise. She had left school at 14 and started work at a biscuit factory in Dublin. Aged 16, she and her younger sister were torn away from their lives and shipped over to London, where their mother (Helen) set up a boarding house for Irish navvies. This was in the '50s, and times were hard for a woman raising two daughters alone. Bed, breakfast, and evening meal for £1 a night. Helen did all the cooking and cleaning by herself. Hardly surprising that there may not have been a great deal of time left to monitor the emotional well-being of two lively teenage girls.

By the time Helen became 'Nanny' to me, she had probably mellowed quite a bit, but she had a reputation for being quick to anger. Nonetheless, she was my 'safe space' and the person I would run away to (I ran away quite a bit). I often heard the story of how she had punched a nun at a Catholic school in Dublin. As a child, my mother was very poorly with Scarlet Fever. When she finally returned to school, she made some mistakes in a lesson, and the teacher made her kneel in the corner (Ah, nuns.... Such beacons of compassion in a school!) Having been forced to stay there all afternoon, she eventually passed out. When Helen found out what had transpired, she was not one to pull her punches

(literally). She flew into the classroom, roaring and furious, and socked Sister Whatsit in the eye. There was no more kneeling after that (well, not in school). There were many more anecdotes about her 'feisty temper,' including the time she found out that her husband had been 'carrying on' with her neighbour. She dragged the hussy down the street by her hair, despite the desperate pleas of the local Garda to "let the poor woman be". Helen was beyond hearing and violent in her rage (woman scorned incarnate). There was much scrabbling around in the dust and a black eye or two (possibly for the policeman also). I can see where my mother inherited her penchant for regulating her emotions with violence. This incident precipitated Helen's move to London, where she lived until she finally shuffled off her mortal coil aged 97 (probably kicking and screaming as she was dragged into the light!). She was a lifelong attender of Mass, and when she could no longer walk, the priest would visit her to offer Holy Communion or hear her confession. In her later years, I went to see Nanny in the hospital, and on one occasion she whispered loudly that the priest was trying to have sex with her. I know there have been a lot of scandals and horrendous abuse associated with the clergy over the years, but I feel this might not have been quite true.

She did return to Ireland on occasion throughout her life, most notably for her ex-husband's funeral, when she

removed her shoes and literally danced on the fresh earth atop his grave. She used to tell me these tales while sitting in a green armchair, cackling away and chain-smoking. She was the youngest of fourteen children and blackmailed her brothers into sharing their cigarettes with her (behind the outdoor lavy) when she was nine years old. She reluctantly stopped smoking at the age of 97, at the behest of the Grim Reaper. Throughout her life, she seemed to relish the idea of people being frightened of her wrath. In her hazy living room, the velvet 'suite' (settee and two matching armchairs) was artfully bedecked with smoke-tinged antimacassars. Shiny pictures of Jesus beamed from the flocked wallpaper, His eyes watching your every move (Benevolently or judgmentally, depending on the day). A dusty plastic container shaped like St Bernadette filled with holy water from Lourdes nestled next to a half-empty bottle of 'Three Barrells Brandy' on the mantelpiece. A familiar yet uncomfortable hybrid atmosphere of love, religion, and righteous anger simmering below the surface. Confusing, but still my place of safety.

But back to the agony of family Christmases. The women in my family liked to do everything 'hard': work, play, hit, and especially, drink, so by lunchtime, the booze had been flowing freely since 11 am, and my mum would cajole, beg, and finally command that I stand up

and 'entertain' everyone. The crippling pressure to perform caused pains in my stomach, and even thinking about it now makes me feel like throwing up. I was just not naturally someone who liked to 'show off'. I loved playing games and pretending to be other characters but standing up and singing as myself felt like a hideous punishment. I lived inside my imagination and escaped to a fantasy world whenever possible. I loved to read books and write stories. An introvert in the middle of a gang of extroverts, like an antelope hanging out with a clan of hungry hyenas. Eventually, I would do my best, usually with my mum saying afterwards, "She does it much better than that at home". Then she would stand up and give her version of "Danny Boy". She really was the natural performer of the family… she always wanted everyone to look at her and applaud and tell her how wonderful she was. I guess she had her own self-worth issues. I also loved performing, but in a different way. I was an actor at heart and wanted to inhabit the skin of a different character. From inside someone else, I was happy to shine. As for me, I was scared of being judged and found wanting. Which would confirm my feelings of not being good enough. I can't remember a time when I ever felt good enough as a child.

In my family, you were always either in favour or out in the cold, and you had to pick a side. Feuds were the norm, and they could sometimes last years. I learned that

to be loved and accepted, I needed to be all things to all people. My relatives were not physically demonstrative, and I discovered that 'achieving things' raised the likelihood of people offering me affection, so every winning rosette and certificate came with added rewards. If I had done something that displeased my mother, she would withdraw affection completely, even going as far as not speaking to me for days at a time. This was agonising and far worse than any physical punishment. I had no siblings; my parents had split when I was one, and I knew nothing about my father. My mum had many secrets in her past, and this was one she was not prepared to share with me.

I remember sitting on my bed one day, around six years old, pondering what was wrong with me and if I was broken somehow. I had a little white shelf in my bedroom (I called it the 'Ballet Corner') with books on famous dancers such as Margot Fonteyn and Rudolph Nureyev, plastic containers with mini point shoes, and fuzzy felt ballet figures in tutus. Sat on top was my prized 'Ballet Sindy'. I had wanted one for years, and when Father Christmas eventually made good, I was devastated to discover that she had broken ankles, and I couldn't put her in a proper 'arabesque.' She sat astride my shelf with her wobbly charity shop feet hanging at strange angles. Useless at ballet but surprisingly good at listening (a bit like me, as it turned out). The way I saw

the situation was this: Parents were meant to love their children, but clearly, my father didn't love me (or he would have shown up at some point), and my mother only loved me if I was winning something or performing.

Most of the time, I was just an irritant in her life, to be tolerated, shouted at, or ignored at will. I was quite pragmatic about it, and my conclusion was this: If my parents didn't love me for being me, I probably needed to try doubly hard for other people to like or love me. I would swing from feeling heartbroken to practical strategy planning mode, depending on the day. I read a lot of Enid Blyton, and the kids were always great at problem-solving, so I took a leaf out of their books. This plan seemed to work well for a long time, and for many years, I lived like a chameleon, changing my colours to fit in with each environment and altering my accent to be accepted. Because of drama lessons as a child, I spoke quite 'well' but roughed up my accent at school. Otherwise, I was called posh and stuck-up. I didn't have the right clothes or shoes to fit in (as we couldn't afford them), so I would also pretend I didn't know things in class or do badly in an assignment on purpose, as I wanted to be liked and not be thought of as a 'goody, goody show-off'.

When I was seven, my mum married again, I think for the second or third time, but I am not quite sure.

There is a lot of mystery about her past. I found a black and white picture in a suitcase, with her clearly getting married to someone. To this day, I have no idea who he is. So, this time, I had a stepdad for three years. It was hard to adjust to a third person in the house. He had no idea how to relate to a 7-year-old, and I had no idea how to relate to a man who was suddenly telling me what to do. I felt left out and angry much of the time, as my mum now focused all her attention on this exciting new relationship. I guess this is a fairly normal way of responding when little care is taken during the family integration. Looking back now, it is interesting that I hated my mum's obsessive smothering, but the opposite (being ignored and dismissed) was equally uncomfortable. There was no balance or harmony, as everything was always extreme. Unsurprisingly, the novelty of a husband soon wore off for my mum, and she soon stopped playing the loving wife role.

Following her usual pattern around new people, she decided she couldn't stand him after all, and their relationship soon became a battleground. As their relationship quickly started to disintegrate, it meant a temporary reprieve for me. Someone else could be on the receiving end of the shouting for a change. I was back in favour as her ally. He was a simple man, probably caught unawares in the beguiling web my mother could spin when she put her mind to it. He was kind to me (I

think), but I resented his presence and the attention he got from my mum. I guess for me, some attention was better than no attention. I really hadn't wanted a stepfather. I had wanted a dog.

By the time I was 10, my stepdad had been thoroughly chewed up and spat out by my mum and had consequently beaten a hasty retreat as far away as possible (sensible decision). My life, however, was about to take a turn for the better. I was accepted at the newly established 'Laine Theatre Arts' dance school in Epsom, Surrey. The principal (Miss Laine) spotted something in me, and although I wasn't aware of it at the time, she soon awarded me a scholarship, which allowed me to carry on dancing when my mum could no longer afford the classes. I later became a "semi-student," attending dance, drama, or singing classes every evening after school, plus on Saturday mornings. Some of my friends from dancing class came from wealthier homes, and when I visited their houses, my posh voice came back into action. My mum had certainly drummed good manners into me, so I was grateful for that.

Well-meaning parents would offer to lend me their daughter's outfits for competitions and auditions. I couldn't see their kindness then; all I felt was SHAME. I was ashamed that people looked at me with pity, and it was a searing, burning feeling that made me feel ugly inside. Although I had a natural talent in all the dance

and drama classes and wanted to shine, I also wanted to blend in and hide. If I stood out too much, I was fearful that people would scrutinise me more closely, and then they might see that I was defective and unlovable. I tried to hide my talents, but in the end, I did it so thoroughly that it got to the point where I could no longer find them, and I didn't believe I was good at anything at all. I was my own worst critic. By now, I had started to dread competitions of any kind.

Unlike the little child feeling the sunshine glow of praise and warmth when I won, now it meant other people might look at me with cold jealousy. Dance school mums can be extremely competitive, way scarier than a bunch of pubescent girls at school, and that is saying something! Sometimes, I won awards and scrutinised the expressions in the eyes of the other kids and parents, looking for judgment and waiting to be 'punished' in some way. It was excruciating for the overly sensitive child I had become and exhausting, trying to second-guess how each person would respond in any given situation. Hypervigilance and anxiety at such an early age. It was such a dichotomy. I wanted to do well, but also wanted to be loved for who I was, not what I could do.

So, how (you may quite rightly ask) did such a reluctant performer end up having a career on the stage that spanned more than 25 years? Despite my misgivings

and fear of 'showing off', I discovered that I did actually love being on the stage, after all. Something inside me lit up when I saw the world through someone else's eyes, and I felt fulfilled. When I was playing a role, I was completely immersed in it and felt unbroken. I was enough.

I particularly loved bigger theatres, where the audience was a warm and welcoming blur, and I didn't accidentally make eye contact and bring myself crashing back to reality. I needed to lose myself in the magic of the show and the character, the dance, or the song. I also loved being part of a company, all working together. As an only child, this connection was blissful to me. In the theatre world, I found a tribe I could belong to. Creative individuals, many of whom had personal issues of some kind that they were struggling with, but came alive on stage. The stories from the 'theatre years' would make a very juicy book on their own (with trigger warnings galore!). Still, I just want to take a moment to thank the amazing people I trod the boards with, in shows such as CATS, Grease, Sunset Boulevard, Taboo, The Beautiful Game, West Side Story, Slice of Saturday Night and Brighton Rock, as well as two of the most memorable theatrical experiences ever (not always for good reasons!); Romeo and Juliet the Musical and Moby Dick: A Whale of a Tale. Talented, hard-working people, many of whom do not get enough credit for their craft,

resilience, and ability to face disaster, get up and start all over again. Musical theatre people, I salute you!

While submerged in the theatre world, I took a brief stroll down one of the darker avenues. I discovered there were other ways to feel good about myself when I was introduced to the dubious pleasures of recreational drugs. Apparently, not all genies lived in glass bottles; some came in little wraps of powder or inside pills. A very fast way to feel good temporarily, and bad for a long time afterwards. Before long, I also learned that some paths were better to get off fairly quickly if you wanted to stay in one piece. Unfortunately, some stayed on those paths for too long and never found their way out of the woods. My heart is with them and the friends and families they left behind, feeling lost, angry, and helpless. And terribly sad.

So, a wild and wonderful tribe of people, drawn together through passion, talent, creativity, and sometimes pain. Dysfunctional though it may have been, I had found a new family.

3

Windmills of Your Mind

Throughout my childhood, Mum would decide every few years that it was time to move house. In the 1970s and '80s, council house exchanges were quite common, with people advertising their current home and what they were looking for instead, a bit like a bigger version of 'Multi-Coloured Swap Shop' on a Saturday morning, but without Noel Edmunds, or Philip Scofield in a closet with a gofer. I never knew what would instigate Mum's urge to move house; maybe she thought happiness would just lie somewhere else, and the grass would really be greener in a different square of terraced garden. I often only got a few weeks' notice that it was time to start the packing procedure again, and my heart would sink. Each move meant a new school and

beginning from scratch to try to fit in. (Time to dust off the chameleon suit again.) During secondary school, we moved three times, once whilst studying for my 'O' Levels. As it transpired, this meant moving from a rather bitchy all-girls school to a great mixed comprehensive, where I was much happier, thanks to my wonderful friend there (Jude), who took me under her wing from day one (no-nonsense, arty and a cynical wisdom beyond her 15 years!). Each time we moved house, we would have to cart all the tea chests and 'stuff' from the previous move (some not yet unpacked), plus all the newly acquired things, so each subsequent house would be fuller than the last. Hoarding really is a terrible condition. No matter how much space or how many rooms you have, they gradually get filled. The same level of importance is attached to everything, be it a diamond ring that belonged to your grandmother or a pile of old newspapers from 10 years ago. I was so used to living in overwhelming clutter that I was always amazed to go to a friend's house and see that they only had just one of everything (I found five food mixers in a bedroom once, and my mother didn't even cook). When I asked why she had bought them, she said it had been such a bargain that she couldn't resist. Items would often be broken, and she would be convinced that she had just the right screw to fix it. If only she could find it!

On a serious note, hoarding is heartbreaking to witness, and as this is my 'memoir' (not my mother's), I won't go into too much detail other than to reflect that she seemed to equate having 'things' with having love. It was a distressing cycle to experience: the euphoria at the initial find and purchase, the dawning realisation that there was nowhere to put it (or it was broken), and then the resignation when it was added to another pile or box, possibly not to be seen again for many years. Then, feeling low as the cycle begins again. I always swore I would not repeat this pattern, but I see it creeping in, albeit on a smaller scale. For me now, it is the endless piles of books I don't have time to read and the ever-growing supply of new crystals (well, there is always another one that just *speaks* to you!). Now that I have arthritis in my toes, my fancy shoe collection has dwindled, only to be superseded by my handbag collection, which is starting to spread to every room. Is it ok because these are expensive 'luxury' items, or is it really just the same as my mum: another form of addiction and another way to try and fill the emptiness inside and feel good enough? What is this need for 'more' of everything, and is it surprising that this would also apply to alcohol?

I left school at 16, clutching my eight O-levels around me like armour. Part of me longed to continue academically and see how far I could go, but a bigger

part recognised that my career path had already been cast in stone since I was four. I got a grant from the local council (they used to offer these for free in those days!), and I bravely strode forth into the next three years of training as a musical theatre performer. My time at Laine Theatre Arts was absolutely fantastic; Exhausting, exhilarating and challenging both physically and emotionally. It was fascinating witnessing so many performers gathering together from different corners of the world, each a big fish in their little pond, now all thrown in together with the sharks. It was good training in resilience for a career in the theatre; you had to REALLY want it to get through the three years with your passion (and limbs) still intact. Not everyone did

As I reached my late teens and began socialising more, I sometimes felt cripplingly shy, even with people I knew. I was confident when performing, but outside of the studio or theatre, I felt as though I had lost my compass. I was so busy trying *not* to be the person my mum wanted me to be that I had lost sight of who I actually was. I felt very gauche, stuck as a confused child in a fully-grown body. I expect many teenagers feel the same nowadays, but somehow, I think we were all a bit more naïve back in the '80s. I soon found that alcohol was the perfect solution to this feeling of being 'other'. Before meeting friends in town, I could buy a can of wine at the 'offie' and drink it on the bus. By the time I

reached the pub or nightclub, I was in just the perfect state of calm and confidence and could avoid the anxiety of the first hour when I felt I didn't fit in and wasn't as cool or trendy as anyone else. I was hyper-sensitive and painfully embarrassed about having less money to spend than other people. The reality was that most of us students didn't have tons of money, but many came from wealthier homes, so it didn't seem to be such an all-encompassing issue for them (My grant covered tuition mainly, so I worked a Saturday job in a hardware shop to fund my social life). Most other students had already flown the nest and were testing their wings whilst staying in shared houses, while I was still at home with my mum. I knew if I was ever 'late,' my mum would be standing at the front door waiting to fight with me or, even worse, she would have locked me out. With this at the back of my mind, my socialising always began on a tense note.

After a drink or two, I no longer felt that I didn't fit in. I relaxed and felt amazing. I could be funny and a bit wild, and people seemed to like this alter ego I could adopt. I became like a weird comic book character; 'Good Michele' by day, who worked hard and quietly behaved herself (like a good Catholic girl should!!), and 'Bad Michele' by night, who threw caution to the wind, had fun, and completely parked her heavy cloak of guilt for the evening (only to have it engulf her totally in the

cold light of day). I had no superpowers other than the heady (and addictive) twin strengths of freedom and confidence.

All it took was three glasses of wine.

Living at home whilst at college was also difficult to negotiate in other ways. The more I tried to assert my independence, the more the extremities of my mother's hoarding escalated. She had limited funds and rather dubious taste, so our house was always filled to overflowing with boxes and black bin liners of odd clothes, dodgy electrical devices, and plastic knick-knacks, mostly bought from charity shops. The wardrobes strained at the hinges and spewed their contents gleefully: Evening dresses and pointy shoes that my mum had kept from her younger years, "just in case I might be able to wear them again one day" (Very " Whatever Happened to Baby Jane"). Even now, in her 80s, she still has clothes from her 20s that she refuses to get rid of. Each new pile of 'stuff' was artistically balanced upon boxes and boxes that hadn't been unpacked from our previous house moves, so if we had a 'spare bedroom' in a house, it was impossible to enter it without being smothered in a falling pile of mangy, moth-eaten coats. I was ashamed of my home and lusted after the friends' houses I visited, where you could walk through the hall and actually turn around at the end instead of having to moonwalk backwards the way you

came. If two people tried to pass each other in our hallway, one would need to try and flatten against the wall, and this would result in garish pictures of crying boys and half-naked mermaids toppling from their precariously placed nails and crashing on top of you, while black bin bags wrapped themselves around your ankles, taking you down like rugby players. It was a dangerous endeavour. "Can't we just get rid of some of this stuff?" I would bellow, feeling frustrated and bruised. "It will come in handy one day," was my mum's reply as she lovingly piled all the crap back up. This home was not conducive to inviting friends over, so it remained a lonely place for me. There were so many 'things', but they didn't seem to bring happiness. Maybe finding just the right object would do the trick? Maybe we were both looking in the wrong places… my mother externally and I internally, but neither of us was happy with what we found there. Neither of us felt good enough. Round and round we went with our individual self-destructive lonely patterns, like two dinghies bobbing helplessly in the vast open sea… aware of one another but unable to help or connect with each other. Circles, patterns, and spirals. Claustrophobic. Trapped.

4

No Business Like Show Business

There were, however, some good memories from my childhood, and many of them were made whilst 'treading the boards.' I started performing on stage at the age of four and continued until I was forty. The theatre was always my magic place of happiness to escape to when reality was too painful. I played a variety of odd little parts at the start, namely a dirty little mudlark (?!) and Dick Whittington's Cat's Girlfriend (also a cat, but white, and a little bit pointless to the story). From there, I progressed to giving noteworthy performances as a sparkling diamond and a monkey in my first Pantomime, "Sinbad," at The Thorndike Theatre in Leatherhead, Surrey. It was my first professional engagement, for which I received the princely sum of £1 per

performance, plus free grub in the Green Room cafeteria (I was ten years old and could eat as much as I liked, so this was the perfect gig!). Next came a few TV adverts, including one for Jacob's Biscuit Selection. This required me to play the daughter of the landed gentry and ride a horse for two days. I was told from an early age to "always say you can do anything" in an audition, so I duly said I could ride. In fact, I didn't know one end of a horse from another, so it proved to be a very uncomfortable weekend (bottom-wise). I did get paid to eat a shedload of lemon puffs, though, so it was worth every bruise.

Life went on, as it does.... School, dancing, acting, singing, and a bit of homework when I could squeeze it in. When I was fourteen, I was in the bath one morning when my mum shouted through the door, "We are going to see your father today". It was the first time she had mentioned him unprompted, so it was a bit of a shock! I remember feeling excited but also very worried (a distinctively unpleasant bubbling in my stomach that would become very familiar later in life when my stage fright started to kick in). It was a moment that I had fantasised about and hoped would happen *one day,* but now that it was here, I wasn't ready. We stood waiting nervously at the front door and watched as a clean, green, shiny car pulled up. A suave, unseasonally tanned man got out and waved. It was a cloudy day, but he wore

sunglasses. And he had a limp. He opened the car door for my mum, who practically batted her eyelashes as she tittered behind her invisible fan ("Bridgerton"-style). I stared in fascination. This was a side of her I didn't recognise. I sat in the backseat, straining for a look at this exotic stranger in the rear-view mirror. Inside, the car smelled artificially fresh… a dangly bit of cardboard wafting its sickly stench in the breeze as he opened the window to blow smoke out. I thought that was very genteel. I was used to sitting in a car where you took a deep breath before getting in and then hoped for the best as you coughed and spluttered in the smoky fug till the journey's end. Second-hand smoke wasn't a thing to be concerned about much in those days. Mind you, neither was firsthand smoke.

I noticed that this stranger had a slight impediment with his 'Rs', as I did. When he eventually removed his sunglasses, I saw my own nutty brown eyes reflected back at me. So, this was my dad.

He was an earthy yet sophisticated sort of man. Ex-army, disciplined in many ways, but very fond of the good life, especially fine food and wine. I didn't see him often, as he lived Northwest, and we were Southeast. In London, that divide is like a chasm. I remember him coming to watch me in a pantomime that first Christmas after we had met. I can't remember when I had felt so proud as I peeped through the curtain and, for the first

time ever, had not one but two parents in the audience. I rushed out of the stage door afterwards, eager to hear his thoughts, and overheard him talking to my mother: "She could do with losing a bit of weight, couldn't she?" he whispered loudly. I had recently won rave reviews in a local paper for my role in the show (playing a Welsh mouse as part of a Flanagan and Allen double act, with a cat called Satan, no less!), but *that* was his comment. Too fat. Great. My heart sank, and I wished I could disappear. I was 14 years old and size 8-10. My mum preened as she lit another cigarette and basked in the perfection of her skinniness. I remember starting to loathe my body at that point, wanting to be a little girl again so my dad would think I was good enough, too. How I wish I could go back to that young girl and tell her she was perfect exactly as she was.

Over the years, my father and I saw each other now and then, and he wrote to me on blue paper, always enclosing a cheque. When we met, he would bring a box of seashell chocolates, and I was scared to eat them in case he commented on my weight again. He would sometimes take my mum and me out for a meal, which was both exciting and stressful. He would eat heartily with great relish, and I would nibble at my food, trying to look thin, whilst my mum ate nothing, just smoked. She must have been ravenous, as she would gorge on toast when we got home. By the age of 21, I had known

him for seven years but had never spent more than a couple of hours alone with him. We decided to have a whole weekend together at his house, just the two of us. We talked about buying property (he owned an estate agency), and he showed me his collection of 'vintage' die-cast pencil sharpeners in the shapes of canons, cars, and planes. They were beautiful, war-like miniatures, each with its place on the shelf: collection, not clutter (fine line!). I really liked them. He cooked wearing a safari shirt and a blue and white striped apron, and we drank plenty of wine. He was more of a Black Tower/Liebfraumilch man than the dry white I preferred, but when in Rome! Then, he played the accordion for me. He used to play it professionally as part of the "Freddy Rossi Trio". To this day, I never pass a street busker playing the accordion without offering some money. It reminds me of a happy time. He told me about when his tank was blown up in WW2 and how he lost part of his leg and was carried to safety by German soldiers. (He had to wear a built-up shoe for the rest of his life.) He also shared a little of his side of the story of my birth and why he wasn't around throughout my childhood. Very different from my mother's 'abandonment' version, of course. I thought this was just the start of us getting to know each other. I had no idea this was the last time I would ever see him.

A few days later, I went 'up north' to spend a season slapping my thigh as Principal Boy in "Mother Goose" in Billingham. I stayed in a grey, soulless building opposite the Forum Theatre. Forbidding-looking but handy for those cast members who didn't drive. It was nicknamed "Colditz" (anyone who has played there will know the one I mean!). I had a single room with a bed, a table, a rickety chair, and a kettle. There was a tiny kitchenette with an unreliable fridge and a microwave. My meals mainly consisted of cream crackers with cheese and pot noodles. No television and, of course, way before mobile phones or the internet. There were ominous clangs as people slammed their doors for the night and firmly turned the keys in the locks (Probably not metal cell doors, but in my memory, they were!) It was not a joyful existence. The night I got back home in January, my grandma called to tell me my dad was dead. No one had even told me he was ill. I guess they didn't want to distress me while I was away working. He never mentioned it when I saw him, although he had looked slimmer. I thought he had just cut down on the puddings. He had always been a heavy smoker and had developed lung cancer, which had spread very fast. From the time he was finally diagnosed to his death was a mere eight weeks.

I was absolutely shell-shocked by his death. I had only just got used to him being alive. I was living with

my first serious boyfriend then, and our relationship was already falling apart. We had been living in a little cottage in Luton, playing at being grown-ups. Although quite wealthy, he had just been caught stealing from the company he worked for. 'Because it was so easy' was his excuse when I asked him why. Final nails in coffins all around. My world felt unsteady beneath my feet, and I didn't know what to do. Once again, I felt trapped and claustrophobic. A theatre friend dragged me along to an audition for a new show called "Sherlock Holmes- The Musical". I have no recollection of it and didn't get the part, but out of the blue, I received a call from Cameron Mackintosh's office (Major West End Theatre producer, for anyone not in the biz). They were taking the show "CATS" on tour for the first time and were still looking to fill one role ('Demeter'); would I be interested in coming along for a private audition? I was mystified. I had never even seen 'CATS', let alone auditioned for it. I thought it was all about amazing balletic dancers, and I knew I wasn't that. The next few weeks were surreal. Chrissie Cartwright was the person in charge of casting the show and had been on the audition panel for Sherlock, so it was she who had spotted me. I was out of shape and certainly too overweight for Lycra (what's new!), but I could sing the Sh*t out of "Macavity", so Chrissie's assistant (Kim Winfield) spent a week working with me at Pineapple Studio in London. I have never

worked so hard in my life, learning the choreography by day and crying my eyes out, grieving for my dad by night. By the end of the week, I wanted that role more than anything on earth. I had done everything I possibly could, and Kim had quite honestly worked miracles. On the final 'judgment day', Chrissie sat and watched me put through my paces, as I sang and danced my little heart out. The next day, I had a phone call from the office, and the part was mine. (Thank you, Chrissie and Kim)

Rehearsals were due to start at Sadler's Wells almost immediately, and then, a few weeks later, we were off to sunny Blackpool to open the show at The Winter Gardens. Early on in rehearsals, the tour cast had a group visit to watch the current London version of CATS. I almost passed out with horror in my seat, agog at the amazing talent of the performers, especially of the person playing my role. 'YOU ARE NOT GOOD ENOUGH,' my brain started yelling. 'I KNOW,' I yelled back. But I did it anyway, and that show, the people, and the tour changed my life.

After a year on the road, playing Blackpool, Edinburgh, and Dublin, I returned to London and sublet a little flat in Wood Green (proper North of the river and well out of my comfort zone) I started in my first West End role at The New London Theatre on Drury Lane, (now called the Gillian Lynne theatre, after the phenomenal choreographer of CATS). Once again, I

was playing the role of "Demeter" (which I was to reprise again several years later). I was 'free' and earning decent money, and I couldn't believe the choices available to me in the big wild world. Having disposable income was still a new experience, and I started to get carried away with buying beautiful NEW THINGS to surround myself with… all the new paraphernalia I had never been able to afford before, shoes, clothes, handbags, and makeup—quality, expensive things. Although I suspected that I was seeking stability and self-worth in material things (just like my mum), it felt so good to be able to choose for myself and discover my tastes. Since leaving home, I felt I could finally breathe freely, without the clutter and second-hand smoke choking me on every side.

Working in theatre was a fabulous life in many ways, but there was definitely also a shadowy side to it. There was often a fair bit of inappropriate behaviour from older directors, producers, and actors. I certainly had my share of unsolicited advances. There was one memorable show where the director took a shine to me and invited me out to dinner to 'discuss my career'. When I very politely said no to the extra 'coaching' he was offering, he fired me the next day in front of the whole cast on stage in the middle of a rehearsal. I remember the company manager rolling his eyes and sighing as he went to smooth over the situation. I was

reinstated fairly swiftly, but it was all very dramatic at the time!

Once I was busy in my career, working full-time in the West End (or on tour around the UK), the amount of socialising and partying (and drinking) was somewhat dictated by the type of show and the part I was playing. CATS was an extremely demanding show in every way, but on the tour, most of us were young and could easily handle a night full of tequila shots and a matinee the next day. Once in the London cast, I had to drive home after performances, so this was always a great gig for sobriety, especially when I went back into the show again at the ripe old age of 27. My early 20s were actually very good times in many ways, even if I didn't fully appreciate them then. I had one great part after another, was busy and happy, and felt the most fulfilled I ever had.

By contrast, there were other shows where alcohol was certainly part of the 'ritual' before, during, and after the performance (I remember one dressing room where we had a wine box next to the water cooler!) In many environments, alcohol was just intrinsically accepted as par for the course backstage.... Champagne in the interval, a quick gargle with Port before going on, or a bottle of vodka and some cans of Red Bull in the fridge to keep you going. In one show, we had a cocktail bar set up in a dressing room, as many of the cast 'died' early in the performance, so we ended up having a social jolly

during Act 2! As long as you didn't mess up on stage, blind eyes were usually turned. By now, I had worked almost continuously for twenty years and was starting to feel exhausted in every way. I still enjoyed being on stage, but the alcohol I was using to control my newly developing performance anxiety started to have an impact. It affected my singing voice and my memory for lines, so much so that eventually, I started to experience panic attacks before going on stage.

Alcohol was such an accepted and integral part of my life that I didn't understand it was the cause of my panic attacks, as it also seemed to be the remedy. I could never have guessed that it would eventually stage a complete takeover and almost ruin my life.

5

Soulmate

Back in my career's halcyon days, in many ways, I was living the dream. When my father died, he left me some money (as well as a beautiful Buddha statue), and once back in London after my CATS tour, I very sensibly used it to get a mortgage and buy my flat. In those days, it was still possible to buy property in London if you looked for bargains, and I found a beautiful two-bed Victorian flat in West Norwood (Southeast London) for a mere £63,000. I had many happy years there: great theatre jobs, fun flatmates, lovely boyfriends (and some not so lovely, as it turned out). I started to believe that I might be ok as a person, and bobbed along quite happily, but somehow, even with friends or in relationships, I felt lonely. The darkness was lurking way beneath the surface; I just refused to see it as I kept my head well above the murky

water and danced and sang above the footlights. 'TTA' at all times! (Teeth, tits, and Ass!) It felt like I had an old pirate treasure chest tied to my ankle with a rusty chain. It was slowly dragging me down. Inside the chest, I kept a big book inscribed with all the shadowy things in my life so I wouldn't have to deal with them. Problems from childhood, tick, maternal abuse, tick, no father, then father, then dead father, tick tick, tick. Falling in love seemed a good way to stay in the light. Still, somehow, I was often drawn to the darkness in others, culminating in a very frightening relationship with a violent sociopath. "Change course", my 'inner safety dial' screamed at me, so I dated a series of nice, kind, non-psychopathic people. But 'Bad Michele' inside was tapping her toes, twiddling her thumbs, and rolling her eyes. "Bor-ing," she sang, "Where's the drama, the adventure, the Jeopardy???"

So, I put my fingers in my ears and said, "La La La, I can't hear you," and worked harder. Maybe if I could envision my perfect boyfriend, I could draw him to me. I realised I wanted a fairytale that wouldn't lead me down a dark path in the woods to a gingerbread house of death (a bit dramatic, but not far off the plot on one occasion). It wasn't exactly like "Witches of Eastwick" spell time, but I decided to start visualising my ideal partner. He would be tall, dark, and handsome (who doesn't love a good cliché?!). He also needed to be emotionally stable,

intelligent, and good with words. Oh, and have lovely hands. And it would be a bonus if he had a nice family. If I had realised how powerful these sorts of wishes could be, I might have added in filthy rich. And so it was that I summoned

"The Brown-Eyed Man".

I first encountered this 'Adonis' in a salubrious venue called "The Green Room", a late-night theatre haunt just off The Strand. Little did I know that this handsome stranger had actually been watching me from afar for a while (well, from the other side of the auditorium, actually, where he was working in the bar). He had christened me "The Girl in the Cap". I had to wear lots of wigs in the show (Sunset Boulevard), leaving me with crazy pin-curled hair when I took them off, so I whacked a black cap on each night before leaving the stage door and heading to the pub. My best pal Daph, aka "Owl Lady" (as she was quite wise and liked to stay up late), and I shared a love of fine wine (or any wine) and did not generally hold back with our consumption. The Brown-Eyed Man had a wingman, too (let's call him "Wilson"). We quickly all hit it off, which led to several weeks of 'hilarious capers'. Sometimes, we would dress up in disguises, borrowing costumes from our show to meet up on matinee days (raincoats, hats, and sometimes, moustaches, and that was just the girls!). Sometimes, I would find poems left for me at the stage

door. It was a good old-fashioned 'wooing'. It wasn't long before the Brown-eyed Man and I realised we had fallen in love. New Year's Eve 1994, he proposed, just 9 weeks after we had met. It was in the Green Room once again, and we were both plastered, but it was a yes from me. I am fairly sure that he was just as much in love with my two fabulous cats (Oscar and Rudy) as he was with me, but that was ok, as we came as a multi-package. A week or so later, he did the proposal again, down on one knee in the theatre, with his late grandmother's platinum and diamond engagement ring. It fitted like it was made for me. The diamond had a little black flaw in it. Perfect.

By the following year (1995), I was back in "CATS", fully lycra-d up and giving my 'Demeter' for the third and final time. It was ultra-gruelling this time round; I fear a dancer's body seems to age faster than any other. We had planned a beautiful wedding, and with every kick, backbend and knee slide, I was determined to earn enough money to make it happen. In March 1996, I was offered the role of "Rizzo" in the shiny, brand-new original tour of "Grease", starring the lovely Shane Richie. It was due to open at The Opera House in Manchester on 13th May 1996. The only problem was that this lovely big wedding was all planned for 12th May 1996 in London! No problem, we thought! By day, I rehearsed "Grease". By night, I performed in "CATS" and occasionally managed to eat and sleep. I had my

technical and dress rehearsals in Manchester all day Saturday, 11th May, I got a lift home to London in the dead of night and then grabbed 4 hours of sleep before getting up feeling (if not quite looking like) like a zombie bride. In no time, my bridesmaid (Charlie) was thrusting Bucks Fizz at me and wrestling me into my wedding dress. She wrangled me like a nervous thoroughbred as I flustered my way from room to room whilst my Uncle Brian (who was giving me away) paced the flat anxiously, putting his top hat on and taking it off every few steps, like The Mad Hatter on speed. The vintage Rolls-Royce pulled up outside, elegant and shiny, and we piled in, ready to tear down to Kent at a rate of knots, given that we were already likely to be fashionably late. This did not go to plan.

I hadn't realised that the vintage-ness of the car also meant it had a top speed of around 40mph. We pootled along like royalty doing a state visit, waving at gawping passers-by. "Lean forward," I muttered through my demure and bridely smile, "it might make the bloody thing go a bit faster". We finally rolled up to the stately home to a round of applause and a few sneaky glances at watches. There was a long day ahead to be enjoyed or endured, depending on your age and temperament. I hadn't seen my fiancé since the day before, but everyone seemed to be smiling, so I assumed he had managed to turn up. My matron of Honour (Daphne) dealt out the

bouquets, and we shuffled into order, ready to march down the aisle. I took a deep breath as the enormous wooden doors were flung open, and we stepped into the candlelit wonder of the "Grand Hall." This amazing space had been the backdrop for many scenes in my favourite film, "The Princess Bride". The sunlight streamed through the ancient windows, and I floated down the aisle, feeling truly happy.

The whole wedding day at 'Penshurst Place' in Tonbridge was joyful; I have the photos to prove it: black and white arty shots of wedding guests racing around the maze, looking sweaty and manic, and a slightly surreal one of the groom playing the violin whilst the bride danced precariously in the shrubbery. I remember very little of the day other than saying, "I do." I wish I could have paid attention to each moment and committed it to memory, but I was so excited, I could barely eat or drink anything. Ironic that on my wedding day, I was probably the only sober adult in the room. The celebrations continued at the Prince of Wales pub on Drury Lane, in London, where we had an evening "do". Happiness and live music with theatre friends, me smiling and hanging onto the wall. Still sober but woozy with exhaustion. Then back to the sumptuous hotel, where we fell asleep for about five minutes before being dragged back awake and driven to the airport to fly back

to Manchester. Then, the final dress rehearsal and opening night of "Grease".

It was an absolutely marvellous wedding, apparently. I just need to watch the video in slow motion one day so I can enjoy it properly. I still have the dress and the shoes in boxes under my bed, neither of which I could get into now. The veil is still doable.

6

Bigger Than the Whole Sky

So, the tour of 'Grease' was a great success, with all the usual excitements and dramas associated with being on the road and away from home and stability. A year or so later, I transferred to the West End cast to recreate my version of "Rizzo" with the London company. I had turned 30 by now, had settled into married life, and we had bought a house together. Eight shows a week playing a role I loved, decent money coming in, safety and security… what more could I want? I was struck in the face by 'Imposter Syndrome', wondering when I would lose that sneaky feeling that I was somehow a fake and not as good as all the other people around me who seemed so sure of themselves. It all seemed a bit too good to be true, and I kept expecting

something to go wrong. Contentment was a new experience for me, and I felt alien and temporary. If I worked harder and harder, then surely one day I would feel properly safe? I was scared to pause too long in case I realised that I still had a hole inside me. I was happy, but warily so, waiting for the other shoe to drop.

Then we got our first dog together, a Bearded/Border collie-cross puppy called 'Ellie'. She brought absolute unconditional love and joy into our lives, and those were some of the happiest days I can remember. She lit up our existence for fourteen years despite suffering from extreme epilepsy for many of them. Animals have always helped me feel so full of love. Caring for them and building trusting relationships often seems easier than with humans.

I had always wanted a big family (having come from such a tiny one), and when babies didn't come along, the stress and disappointment eventually became unbearable. The clock was ticking as I approached my mid-30s, and it became time to get some medical intervention. The IVF cycle can be traumatic in many, many ways: so much hope, so many hormones injected, so much discomfort, and so much heartbreak. I completely stopped drinking alcohol and didn't even notice, so great was my focus on eating healthily, taking all the right vitamins, and preparing for our family. I was bursting with viable eggs, and when two embryos were

implanted, I was overjoyed. I already felt pregnant. I was 100% certain it had worked. I went and bought a pair of baby booties in a leopard print box and hid them in my wardrobe. Two days before the magical test to confirm pregnancy, my dream was shattered. I couldn't believe it… Everything had gone so well. There clearly was something dreadfully wrong with me if I couldn't hold onto an embryo for two weeks. Maybe I had tempted fate by buying the baby shoes? Maybe I shouldn't have been doing eight shows a week at the same time and should have taken to my bed. What I needed was someone to talk to, and I wish there had been a counsellor available to share with and verbally process the agony I was feeling. My husband was equally disappointed, but his way of coping was to file his emotions away in a box and carry on as normal. So, I did the same. I just carried on doing eight shows a week as if nothing had happened. In private, I dealt with my feelings in the only way I knew how… I numbed them by drinking alcohol and tried not to leave a sober gap where the emotions could take hold and tear me apart. They said we could try another IVF cycle in 6 months, but by then, our marriage had started to fall apart as we turned away from one another to deal with our sadness. It was a lonely existence. Bit by bit, I slid down a dangerous and slippery slope on my own. Although I was unaware at the time, this was the start of a

downward spiral that didn't stop until I hit the very bottom with an almighty thud.

During the following months, my new best mate, Sauvignon Blanc, and I started having a right old time. When I was in her company, I always felt strong and powerful and that I could fit in anywhere. She and I had a special relationship without judgment. She didn't mind if I swigged her from a chipped mug, as long as I finished the whole bottle. She really was the most amenable companion for all of life's events.... Had a bad day, have a drink and forget about it.... Got a new job, celebrate with a few drinks... said or did something bad when you were drunk last night, then better have LOTS more drinks, so you don't have to think about it. Open a bottle, and the magical genie pops out to cure all your ills.

This idea of alcohol as a panacea for everything might not be a surprise to many people... I know I was not alone in this culture of thinking that it is only a good night out if you get totally wasted. The drinking is not the accompaniment to the evening. It is the whole point of it. "I am half-Irish after all... surely it is in my blood?" I told myself reassuringly. I had every possible excuse under the sun to justify my alcohol habit. Boozing was no longer something I did to socialise or boost my confidence. Now, I drank at home alone almost every day. I watched the clock carefully and never drank

before midday. That meant I didn't have an 'issue' as I had some control over myself and my life. Oh yeah, baby, who was I kidding?

On the rare occasions I tried not to drink alcohol when out, I remember the teasing and coaxing of other people: "Don't be so boring, have a real drink; you deserve it." So easy to be convinced… 'Yes, you're right, I DO deserve a drink, ' as if it were a reward instead of poison for me. Other people having one or two drinks and saying, 'Right, I've had enough.' But it was NEVER enough for me…I just didn't have a stop button. The alcohol made me feel good (mostly). I didn't want that feeling to end and reality to come crowding back in with all its psychedelic, scary memories. Being drunk was chaotic, but when sober, my life was becoming equally chaotic. I knew something needed to change, but I was not yet ready to face the gigantic elephant in the room.

7

Lions and Tigers and Booze (Oh My!)

As my 40th birthday loomed, I decided to take stock of my life. Maybe I needed a new challenge, and maybe in a different place, I would be a different person…. Aha! (I thought triumphantly) I could be an adventurer and do something to make myself feel proud (in other words, run away). I bought my first-ever rucksack and a ticket to Namibia. I was only going for two weeks, but I had enough stuff to last two years. I always seemed to carry a lot of baggage, but the irony was lost on me at the time. I spent most of the 12-hour flight sitting bolt upright or leaning against a toilet door and holding my breath as much as possible, as my gag reflex was very over-active, especially after several mini

bottles of wine to 'calm my nerves' (I could always find a good reason to drink, wherever I was)

I stayed in a hostel called "Chameleon" on my first night in Africa, which was filled to the rafters with gap-year students and wizened tourists who had seen it all and had the tanned skin of a rhino to show for it. Long after the fresh-faced twenty-somethings had gone to bed, I was still at the bar chatting and 'being sociable'. Only when the last of the oldies had retired did I realise it was just me and an extremely bored barman. I had been having a right old time and, as always, couldn't bear the evening to come to an end. I always had to be last up, as if I was proving a pointless point of some kind.

The following morning dawned too brightly, and I staggered back to the hostel with dark glasses and my cache of supermarket supplies and treats to see me through the next fortnight in the middle of nowhere. This mainly consisted of a large wine box (red, due to the lack of chilling facilities) and an enormous block of something that was trying to pass as cheese. After many bumpy hours in the back of a minibus, we dismounted expectantly and came face to face with a rather startled warthog, who snuffled aggressively at our legs, leaving small abrasions and a trickle of saliva. I discovered in the coming days that warthogs are very pushy, zebras are grumpy and have sharp teeth and baby baboons, are

thieving terrorists by day, and snuggly angels in nappies by night.

I fell in love with Namibia almost from the moment I arrived, but the seesaw of utter joy and daily terror I experienced over the next two weeks challenged me more than I could ever imagine.

Although my first trip to Namibia was just for two weeks, I really wanted to see if I still had any inner strength and adventure left in me. If the person I used to be was still lurking somewhere inside. I was absolutely terrified of spiders, sharing rooms with strangers, feeling like a fat, frumpy old lady amongst a bunch of lithe teenagers, and especially not having enough alcohol. As it happened, none of my fears were much of an issue. It is hard to focus on the little spiders when you are batting away giant flying beetles! Our first morning as volunteers was surreal; sitting in an outdoor classroom and having someone write the daily tasks on the board. What's strange about that, you may ask? Well, my group leader said we had a particular set of animals to care for, which included two adolescent lion brothers, a bunch of baby baboons, and the crocodiles. WHAT?!!!

He took us on a tour of the sanctuary, and if you were an animal lover, you would have felt that you had died and gone to heaven. Admittedly, much of the work was sweeping and cleaning up crap, but at this time, Namibia had granted special licences for certain

volunteers to work closely with wild animals in captivity. We had a short safety induction, signed a piece of paper to say we wouldn't sue if we got eaten, etc, and then off we went. Probably my worst experience was the day they called "Meat Factory." I hadn't eaten meat since I was 21 years old, and could not imagine that this activity would likely be one I would enjoy. It wasn't. We all stood around tables and were given a variety of knives, a chopper-thing, and a saw. There was a squeaky wheel sound as a trolley came round the corner, filled to overflowing with bits of dead animal. (Think Texas Chainsaw Massacre but without the masks). I wasn't sure whether I wanted to be sick or pass out, but I did neither, as I was the oldest one at the table and didn't want to be 'that person' (Like the medical student who faints at their first autopsy). I did cry as I chopped, but the fact remained that the animals had to be fed, and all the local people would bring their dead animals in exchange for a little money, so it was good all round (well, except for the dead animal and us poor sods that had to chop them up!)

I can't say I was enormously enamoured with the two crocodiles from the start either, and I did have a mild panic when we were shown a long stick and told we would have to lean over the little bridge and clean their teeth with it. This, it transpired, was a hilarious joke, and one I was to use myself many times when I later became

a volunteer coordinator. It was certainly the fastest way to see fresh-faced volunteers very quickly need to rush to the loo! With the crocodiles, it was pretty gross, though, as they like to feast on rotting flesh, so we had to throw over extremely stinking meat, which they snuffled at with crocodile glee. This is pretty much the extent of crocodile action in this story, with two exceptions, including the time one big fella managed to crawl out of his 'area' overnight and was discovered (with great horror) in the guest swimming pool! The rescue manoeuvre required a small army of workers, including me, to somehow get the crocodile out of the pool and transport him about 100 feet. One incredibly brave man jumped in the pool with a length of rope, which the croc immediately grabbed hold of. He then went into a 'death spin' and after a few turns, the rope was wrapped around his mouth, tying it shut. More people then leapt into the water and lifted the croc onto the grass at the side of the pool, and ten of us carried him back to the water he lived in (it probably only needed 8, but all of us wanted the opportunity to touch a live crocodile!). This time, the hero of the hour sat on top of the crocodile by his head, while several other volunteers sat on the rest of him to limit the thrashing. 'Crocodile Dundee' took a deep breath and cut the rope before being hauled out super quickly before the croc

realised he was free again. Far too much excitement at 8 am on a Sunday morning!

The other crocodile anecdote was even briefer but equally exciting/terrifying. This was at a baboon sanctuary in South Africa. I was sitting by the banks of the river, enjoying a bite to eat, when somebody spotted a croc heading towards us in the water. "RUN!" she shouted (as if we needed the prompting!), and we did the best Husein Bolt impressions we could manage in flip-flops. Luckily, it was a very hot day, and the croc clearly couldn't be arsed to give much chase once on the land… it was more like a bit of casual sport for him. He ambled off to bask in the sun with the other crocodiles, which was what he was supposed to be doing at midday. I then had a very important lesson from one of the seasoned volunteers: "Next time a crocodile chases you, ZIG ZAG". She said, nodding wisely. "They can run fast in a straight line, but it really slows them down to have to keep changing angles". I will certainly remember that, but I am hoping my crocodile-interaction days are generally behind me.

Back to my first experiences in Namibia, though. Before the rescue centre grew and had its own special 'volunteer village', we used to stay in small wooden huts. My absolute favourite time was when we had a baby baboon sleepover. I would spend as much of the day as possible in the enclosure with the young baboons. They

took a while to trust me, but I knew I had been accepted when they started grooming me or chose to sit on my shoulders on a baboon walk. My favourite baboon was Jacob, who had had his tail chopped off at some point. The baby baboons were all orphans, and some had been kept as pets. Apparently, it was great fun to watch baboons drinking and smoking, so sadly, many of those I worked with in Africa were addicts who were keener to have a cigarette than a piece of fruit. They were all exceptionally naughty and would steal anything you had. Hair scrunchies and sunglasses were a no-no, and woe betide if you had any obvious piercings. Jacob tried to pull a mole off my tummy once. On one sleepover evening, we had gone to the main house and put nappies on the baboons (with little holes made for their tails to poke out), and then we carried them back to our huts, with bottles of formula. The first hour or so was utter chaos, with three baby baboons chasing each other and careering around the room, literally swinging from the curtain poles and light fittings. If you weren't extra vigilant with the nappies, it could be a very messy experience all round. Eventually, the baboons wore themselves out and snuggled up with their 'mama' for the night. I can't say that I got much actual sleep, with a baboon on my chest, holding my finger in one hand and a handful of my hair in the other.

Over the next couple of years, I was back in Namibia another three or four times. It was the perfect escape from my real-world life, and I had fallen in love with everything there. On one visit, part of my chore list was to help raise four baby lion cubs. There had been a recent visit to the sanctuary by Angelina Jolie and, in her honour, the cubs were named Brad, Maddox, Pax, and Knox. In captivity, cubs need to be removed from their parents fairly soon, as the father will often behave in an unfatherly and murderous manner. Part of his 'job' is to assess the area the pride lives in and compare that with the ratio of available food and the number of hungry mouths to feed. Although the lions were very well fed here, the biological urges kicked in, and very often, the male would kill some or even all of the offspring. Consequently, this unbelievably cute foursome needed human intervention and to be taught the lion rulebook until they were old enough to manage without us.

Our 'foster lioness' jobs included feeding the cubs with formula. The baby baboons were great at this when it was their turn, and they would helpfully hold the bottles with their little fingers, but lion paws were less agile, and often the milk would end up everywhere but in the cubs' mouths. After feeding, we had to hold them up and burp them, and then the least fun part, moisten a cloth and rub their bottoms gently to encourage them

to poo. The mama lioness would be using her tongue, but foster parent roles did have their limits!

The sanctuary grew, as did the number of volunteers, from around 15 per fortnight to 50, and I was offered the role of volunteer co-ordinator. One of my jobs was accompanying the volunteers on a 'lion walk' in the Bush. Together with Frikkie (who was the head of the volunteer programme and an amazingly wise 'nature man'), we would round up some volunteers and go to one of the lion enclosures where 'Zion' and 'Trust' now roamed (the young lions I had been chucking meat at the previous year). These brothers were getting bigger now (around 2 years old) and would soon be too mature to interact with volunteers safely. They had been born in the sanctuary and were very well fed, but at heart, were still wild animals. As with many brotherly tales, one lion was very good and one very bad. Friendly Zion came on the walks. Each time, I had to explain the etiquette of being around lions, which had three main rules.

1. Don't bend down.
2. Don't turn your back.
3. Don't run.

Of course, there was always one volunteer who panicked when Zion started nuzzling around their stomach area, who turned tail and started legging it down the track. Zion would flick his ears in amusement and take after the volunteer at a rate of knots. He would then

leap onto their back from behind and fling them to the ground. Once there, he would just get off and amble away nonchalantly. It was the chase that was fun for him. Maybe not so fun for the volunteer (who would certainly have one or two bruises), but hey, it was a great story to tell their friends. With lions, it is always best to play by the rules. There was one day, though, when the rulebook went out the window entirely. This time, I was the one in the hot seat.

I was in the passenger seat of the Baki (truck), and there was a small gang of volunteers in the back, behind the metal dividing screen. They had several buckets of raw meat, as we were to be feeding other lions on the way back. To do this with the big lions, you would grab a donkey leg (or part thereof) and then fling it with all your might so it would fly over the electric fence to the lion. These legs were extraordinarily heavy, so this didn't always go to plan. Sometimes, it hit the fence and flew back, almost taking your head off with the power of the rebound. Occasionally, if it were a different, fleshier cut of meat, it would stay hanging on the top of the fence, tormenting both the thrower and the lion, until we saw which side it fell.

Anyway, on this particular day, all was as usual, and I sat in the passenger seat, waiting for Frikkie to encourage Zion out of the enclosure and into the other truck (sometimes I drove with volunteers sitting behind

me, and sometimes I could see a big hairy lion head in the rear- view mirror!) Suddenly, I heard a panicked shout of "Get back, get back!" and a large amount of scrabbling. The driver's door was wide open, and to my horror, an enormous lion leapt into the front of the truck and onto my lap. His head was next to my head, his enormous paws squashing my thighs. I froze with terror as my panicked brain screamed at me, "You are going to die right now, AGGHHHHHH!" In the distance, I could hear someone shouting: "Don't move" (as if!) and saw the lion jolt a little, as Frikkie tried to pull him out backwards, by his tail. Understandably, the Lion wasn't too keen on this and let out an anguished roar. I could smell hot, foul, meaty breath, and his glinting incisor was right in front of my nose. He had leapt in smelling the meat, thinking he was going to have a sneaky picnic, and now we were both stuck; he with no dinner, except, possibly me. In my moment of frozen terror, something dawned on me. This wasn't "Zion", this was his brother "Trust" who did NOT go on lion walks because he was unpredictable and dangerous.

It is interesting how a person behaves in a traumatic situation, and I became utterly calm, as my heart slowed, and I tried not to breathe. My senses became ultra-sharp, and with my 'Spidey' hearing, I made out a few words, muffled as if under water; "Open the door and slide out." My left hand inched towards the handle, oh so

slowly. As my shaking hand connected with the metal, my heart started to speed up again until I could feel it banging against my chest. Creaking horror film-style, the door of the truck swung open. I inched my bottom across the seat and continued sliding outwards until my foot was on the ground. I took a deep breath, yanked my other foot out, and slammed the door shut.

Meanwhile, Frikkie waggled a big piece of meat frantically, and the lion reversed itself out and chased him back into the enclosure. My legs gave way, and I collapsed onto the sand, propped up against the car like a rag doll. Wow… close encounters with a dangerous lion and not a mark on me. I think even my Guardian Angel must have been sweating by now! Somebody has footage of this drama somewhere in the world, as one of the volunteers was filming from behind. That certainly would have made interesting viewing on YouTube: "This was the day our volunteer coordinator was eaten by a lion". Not one for tourist information promos!

I don't think anyone would have begrudged me a drink after that, or the time I had to run through the wild dog enclosure with several of them screeching behind me, having already been electrocuted on the electric fence ("Fear Factor" day). Or the time in South Africa when a drug-addicted baboon accidentally tore the retina in my eye. He didn't mean to, he was sitting on my shoulders at the time, and another helpful baboon pulled

his tail., So he grabbed the nearest thing to hold onto, which happened to be my eyeball! Lots of 'mishaps' and me like a cat with more than nine lives, yet I was so incredibly happy… dirty, sore, covered in bruises and bites but totally in my element. But I still needed the alcohol at the end of every day, like a soothing balm to take away all my stress, worries, and near-death experiences. I just could not imagine my life without it.

8

Last Chance

I should mention that I did still have a husband throughout all of this (albeit a very unhappy one). His family had tried to be supportive, but I had hurt them all too many times with my behaviour, and they had eventually drifted further away until they were tiny dots in the distance. Before the bitter end, and as an act of final desperation, I had planned a holiday together (always searching for the Emerald City elsewhere). Maybe we could rebuild some of our crumbling foundations in a different place. I wanted to share the magic of my beloved Africa and, for some crazy reason, thought it would be a great idea for my husband and me to embark on an amazing 3-week trip together. We would spend time under the clear, starry night out in the red sands of the Namibian desert, trail along the famous Garden Route and wine-tasting trails of South Africa (oh

dear), culminating in a ten-day volunteer programme at the Cango Wildlife Ranch in Oudtshoorn. What could possibly go wrong?!

By the time we set off to Heathrow airport, we were barely talking, and that was pretty much the state of play for the entire three weeks. There were the occasional alcohol-fuelled screaming matches, but as this was pretty normal for us by now, I hadn't realised at the time that my husband had already decided to call it quits. Halfway across the world wasn't the ideal place to end a marriage, so we ploughed on, desperately 'enjoying' our once-in-a-lifetime holiday. We were part of a small group, stuck together for the whole 3-week experience. The only thing more awkward than a couple not speaking to each other is to stick them in the middle of a bunch of jolly holidaymakers. One extremely memorable day was the 'action-packed adventure experience'. This included zip wires through the jungle, quad-biking through the countryside, and then abseiling down an enormous cliff to a beach. I can't imagine what we were thinking. Neither of us were adrenaline junkies, so it actually sounded like torture, rather than the fun it was professed to be.

The zip wiring was fairly ok, except for a vast amount of chafing and no voice left from screaming. I couldn't get my head around the fact that people do this for fun. To escape from prison, maybe, but otherwise,

not for me. Next, we bounced our way across the countryside to the quad bike place. The instructor was fairly blasé with his instructions, except for the dire warnings regarding tipping up the quad bike. Apparently, this was a very dangerous and expensive thing to do and to be avoided at all costs. There seemed to be simple stop/start mechanisms, and my cunning plan was to go slow so I felt safe at all times.

The cunning plan of everyone else seemed to be to go as fast as humanly possible, and they raced around, whooping with joyous abandon. Bearing in mind this was all on the top of the cliff, I sensibly employed my excellent driving skills and slowed down appropriately as I approached a sharp bend. How was I supposed to know that you needed to go faster around bends with these four-wheeled monstrosities? I almost ground to a halt as I climbed further and further up on the grassy verge, and in slow motion, I felt the quad bike slipping from under me. Yes, I jumped. To my mind, the only thing worse than turning over this expensive hunk of metal was to have it land on top of me. Despite generally feeling crap about myself, I did not want my obituary to say that I had been squished to a pulp at the top of a cliff. There was lots of shouting, and once it was established that I was alive and that the bike was not ruined, everyone soon lost interest as we trooped obediently to the next bit of 'fun':

The Abseiling.

Now, I realise that in most activities, I come off as the idiot who messes up, but finally, FINALLY, I discovered something I could actually do right. What they hadn't specified at the get-go was that this abseiling lark was from one of the highest cliff edges in South Africa down a sheer drop to the sea. Neither my husband nor I had ever done this, BUT I had one advantage in this round of 'The War of The Roses': he was frightened of heights, and I wasn't. His fear was so great that on one of our first-ever holidays together in Turkey, we had gone on a boat trip together. It took him a long time to dive off the side, as it was fairly high, but he eventually managed it. Then we saw all the local lads climbing up a rock and leaping or diving off into the crystal blue ocean. Well, we were still in the first flush of love, and my dear boyfriend (at the time) was filled with an urge to display his manliness and virility. "Get the camera out", he yelled as he followed the twelve-year-old boys up the rock. Yes, you have guessed what happened next. I had the zoom trained on him as the tiny GIRL in front leapt fearlessly into the water. I noticed that my boyfriend had seemed to have turned very pale under his newly acquired suntan. The people in the queue behind him started to get restless. "Come on, come on", I muttered, still poised to catch the perfect moment of his daring feat. Suddenly, he dipped

out of view of my lens. "Has he jumped?" I thought, scanning the water excitedly, waiting for him to pop up, shining in all his glory. Oh no. The next thing I saw was him shoving his way past the now disgruntled would-be divers and then squatting down. He inched his way back down the rock, bit by agonising bit, on his BOTTOM. For him, it was humiliating, but for me, it was the funniest thing I had ever seen. It also made him more human, and I loved him all the more for it.

Now, at this final action-adventure hurdle in South Africa, I had this cheeky card up my sleeve. There were five or six in our group, and one by one they bleated out their excuses as to why they couldn't do the abseil. I peered over the cliff, and my heart nearly stopped at the distance we were supposed to lower ourselves to. My husband took one look and nearly fell over it, in his urgency to back away to safety. One 21-year-old girl looked excited and said she would do it. That left just me then. I looked around at the faces who, quite frankly, were not expecting much of me and said, "Yep, I'm doing it too"

Now you must understand that I didn't want to do it, but it seemed to me that if I did die this way, it was a more heroic ending than the squishy pulp version. I listened very carefully to the instructions and opted to go first before I changed my mind. My husband was watching me with a strange expression. To this day, I am

not sure if it was admiration for my 'bravery' or a crafty calculation about finally getting shot of me. As I lowered myself backwards off the cliff, I muttered to myself, "You can do it, don't give up, just get to the bottom and see what happens next". My hands were shaking so much that I could hardly feel the rope thing that was preventing me from crashing down onto the rocks below. The first 30 seconds were actually ok, as I bounced around on the cliff face thinking," I'm doing it, I'm doing it!". Then my feet reached a ledge, and I decided the safest thing was to stay there until a helicopter came to rescue me. There was much enthusiastic coaxing from above and eventually, I heard a very frustrated South African voice yell "Move your arse! You can't bloody stay on a bloody ledge all bloody day!". Fair enough, I conceded and lunged backwards. As I bounced around in terrifying mid-air and crashed into the rock periodically, I thought again about how strange humans were. Why, oh why, would anyone choose to torture themselves like this? Still, I had a point to make (um, that I wasn't a complete wuss?), so I obligingly swung back and forth, my hands gripping so tightly they were almost frozen like an Egyptian mummy's withered claw. Eventually, I was on the beach, although it was my bottom that found it first. My monster hands wouldn't let go of the rope, so I sat there clutching it, and as the adrenaline slowly started to seep

out of my system, I burst into tears with relief. I wasn't dead, and I had achieved something that others had not dared to do. A weird sensation came over me, warm and glowy. I actually felt proud of myself for the first time in many, many years. I wasn't useless at everything, and what's more, I was grateful to be alive. These feelings and thoughts had been dormant for a very long time, but they were resurfacing. Then, maybe that means there might be something to look forward to.

Climbing back up to the top was almost worse than going down. The route was zig-zagged and obviously less steep, but the lactic acid in my legs from the post-traumatic adrenaline desertion meant I had full-on jelly legs. I wobbled my way up and collapsed at the top as if I had just done Everest. There was a cacophony of 'well-dones', and my husband looked slightly green but pretty impressed. He had videoed my descent with shaking hands. I don't think even the insurance money would have made up for watching me plummet to my death in front of his very eyes! "See", I said bravely, "I am still worthwhile. I have grit and courage, and don't give up". Well, I thought it, at least. My mouth was so dry, my lips were stuck to my teeth in a passable Humphrey Bogart impression. It was time for the final leg of the trip, and the part where I knew I would be in my element: the animals.

Rather than the amazing hands-on experience I had with the animals in Namibia, Cango Animal Park was pretty much an exotic zoo, with cages and strict rules. The staff weren't really sure what to do with their team of expectant volunteers (this was a fairly new programme), so each day they made up some random tasks to keep us occupied and out of the way.

These included:

1. Cleaning out snake cages
2. Making interactive toys for lions
3. Giving bits of fruit to Ring-tailed Lemurs
4. Putting down bowls of meat for baby tigers

WHAT?!!! These jobs were so tame. Where was the jeopardy and wildness? Ah, I realised, maybe I do thrive on a bit of adrenaline, just not the sporty kind. It just felt so boringly safe and barely a step up from being a visitor at the park. In retrospect, I can see I had numbed myself with alcohol for so long that it took quite a lot of extremity for me to feel any emotions, either positive or negative ones. Unfortunately, it came as a package deal: numb the pain, sadness, shame, embarrassment, and fear, but alongside that, you also numb the ability to feel happiness or experience love.

The day spent in the reptile house was not one of my favourites. I didn't have a particular fear of snakes, but in general, I am not drawn to any being that doesn't blink much. I also did a cage dive with a shark; the eyes were

as terrifying as the teeth. The scariest part of all for me was being underwater, and that aroused such feelings of panic I would have willingly ridden the shark back up to the top if I could have breathed the air again. (By the way, this was in a pool, not in the sea a la JAWS-style. I am not totally insane!) The snake keeper was quite a jolly man who enthused about his beloved collection as if they were fluffy puppies. They were all equally unappealing to me, although it was interesting to find out which ones would squeeze you to death and which ones would stab you with life-ending poison. Snake man would remove each one on a special stick, allowing us to clean their cage whilst they watched us from a different cage, glowering with evil snake thoughts. "I need to be quick with this one", he informed us, as he whooshed past, with just a little bead of sweat dripping from his brow. We peered eagerly at the tiny, innocuous snake that was clearly some kind of troublemaker. Snakeman let out a sigh of relief as he brandished his now-empty stick. "That one did THIS", he announced, thrusting his hand in front of my face like a street magician. We all gasped as we saw his deformed half-finger. "Did it bite your finger off?" I whispered, full of awe. "No, of course not, it's a snake," he retorted. "He sank his fang in, and I had to chop my finger off before the poison spread", as if that was any better. The Reptile House Day was one of the longest I can remember. I am sure some people

get off on watching these creatures stand still for hours, but generally, I prefer my animals to have a little bit more oomph and action.

Ring-tailed lemurs were the epitome of oomph and action, and visits to their little 'island' were joyful. We would hold out bowls with a selection of fruit and veg, and they would stretch out their long, nimble fingers, selecting their favourites as thoughtfully as a child choosing from a pic 'n' mix stand. I loved the lemurs, and they confirmed to me that primates were definitely my favourite animal family, just not always the human members.

Moving over to the big cats, our task for the afternoon was to create something for the slightly bored and restless lions to do. 'Enrichment' if you will. We were supplied with paper, string, and safety scissors, like a 'craft afternoon at the 'home for useless volunteers'. Once I had got over myself, I quite enjoyed playing with the bits and bobs, and eventually, we had come up with a large ball and a 'Guy Fawkes '-type figure. The idea was that the lions would kick the ball around a bit and then beat the fella up, much like an afternoon at Mill Wall in London. Proudly, we carried our creations to the bridge overlooking the lion area. Most were asleep in the sunshine (as lions are meant to be at this time of day), but we had toiled away and were determined the lions would wake up to have fun and enjoy their enrichment.

I think my husband was nominated (as the tallest), and he threw down the ball with all his might, gently grazing a lion's head. The lion dutifully lifted it, yawned, and batted the ball away like a fly. Oh well, maybe later, when it was a bit cooler. We decided to get a bit of excitement going with "Bob", our man. We started shouting and jeering, mob-style and caused a bit of commotion so that all the nearby visitors started wandering over to investigate. We waggled Bob over the lion enclosure suggestively, making strange noises that we thought might excite a lion's curiosity. Eventually, one sauntered over, looked up, and opened his mouth in a half-hearted raw-come-yawn. We didn't want to miss the moment, so after a one, two, three, we launched Bob into the lion pit gleefully, like a bunch of people on a day out at the Coliseum. The lion was certainly very surprised, and then his hackles rose. We held our breath expectantly.

The lion looked at Bob calmly, and Bob's squiffy marker pen eyes looked back at the lion. If we had smeared poor Bob in meat juice, we might have got a swifter reaction, but the lion seemed to sigh with resignation. I like to think that he glanced up at us in the posh seats to see which way our thumbs would go, but in fact, he grabbed Bob by the head and shook with all his might. All the hours of screwing up newspaper, paper mâché work, and tying limbs together with string vanished in a moment as Bob's body scattered to the

four corners. After no more than 5 seconds, he was annihilated, and the lion dropped his head to the ground. He couldn't even be bothered to give it a kick for good measure. Enrichment complete, he strolled back to the others, lay down, and went back to sleep. There were a few sniggers and a half-hearted smattering of applause from the visitors, and the volunteers slunk away, avoiding eye contact. Maybe we should have thrown one of the sniggering visitors in and seen some real enrichment. Grrrr.... What a load of old crap!

The final job I can remember at the animal park was feeding the tiger cubs. I was already pretty au fait with lion cubs, but these tigers were about 5 months old and a different kettle of fish entirely. You know when a cat lies on its back and rolls about in a 'tickle my tummy' kind of way and then stabs your hand with its nails as soon as you do? Tigers are just like that, except their paws were almost the size of my face. There were three of them, and they had started to learn some cheeky games, including how to stalk their prey as a tag team. It was beautiful to watch, but being the 'playtime prey' was somewhat terrifying. I had a lot of very large scratches and bruises. None of the other volunteers were up for this job, and the keepers used to stand at the side and laugh at the crazy woman who tried to outthink tigers in tiger games. The truth was I LOVED everything about them, and if that meant a bit of pain here and there, I

was prepared to take it, just to be in their company. Tigers are much more dog-like than other big cats (including enjoying swimming), and somehow, I could connect with them. They were straightforward and didn't mess with you. I just didn't have the right teeth and nails to play their games fully. I loved making the snuffling noise they liked ("Chuffing") and feeling their weight snuggling up to me. Many years later, I was to discover that my Power Animal is a Tiger (If you have worked with Shamanism, you will be familiar with this idea).

It was good that I developed this tiger passion, as it was something to hold onto as my relationship with my husband disintegrated beyond repair, bit by agonising bit. We both knew we would be happier apart at this stage, and I remember walking along a beautiful South African beach, both of us crying as we realised we wouldn't grow old together. It was probably the most honest we had been with each other for a very long time.

Back home, my husband had finally abandoned the sinking ship (like a rat?!) as the waters were now too choppy and he felt he was drowning too. Well, this is how it felt at the time. Looking back, I know he felt he was unable to help me and was, in fact, enabling me in my addictive/compulsive behaviour, so he got the hell out of Dodge while he still could, hoping that might shock me into pulling myself together. (He actually just

moved down the road and rented a room from a stripper…. You couldn't make this up!) I felt, however, that he had abandoned me at my lowest point, and for a while, I felt utterly alone in my pit of despair. I was frightened, as I couldn't see a future for myself. I was also resentful and angry at everyone, individuals, and the whole world in general. I had thought I was a good person, so how had I ended up here? I knew I was almost at rock bottom, but I still couldn't take responsibility for my actions; it was just too painful. Better to blame my parents, my husband, and everyone around me for not loving me enough and letting me fall this far. I was desperate for love, but still did not feel worthy of it.

9

Spinning Wheel

On my final visit to Namibia, things started to take a turn for the worse. Because I only drank in the evenings, my hands shook in the mornings as I suffered withdrawal symptoms. Are you ok, Michele?" Asked one of the bright and bubbly volunteers one morning at breakfast. "Why are you shaking?" "I need caffeine," I growled back. "Don't speak to me until I have had two cups of coffee." I felt ratty much of the time, constantly swinging between drunk at night and stone-cold sober in the daytime. I didn't understand that I was suffering withdrawal symptoms, and in between the extreme states, I chugged endless cups of coffee, trying to feel normal. I was becoming tired of the young volunteers and their endless, energetic neediness, as the role required me to be on duty seven days a week, day and night. I longed for people of my age to have

conversations with, and despite being surrounded by people all the time, I became very lonely. A new volunteer coordinator joined and took the other bed in my hut. I felt very uncomfortable with her as she made jokes about my age and commented on the fact that I had a wine box by the bed. I was shocked; didn't everyone have a glass of wine before bed?? It was the first time anyone had openly mentioned my drinking, although I expect plenty was said behind my back. When we had a campout under the stars, the volunteers would order drinks to be brought in a cold box, usually a beer or two. I would order a beer or two as well, but also a bottle of wine, 'just in case'. This girl was much more on the same wavelength as the volunteers (many were 18/19 years old, and I was 41 by then), and I started to feel vulnerable. People who had been friends and allies for the past couple of years were suddenly ghosting me and hanging out with this new interloper, and it gradually started becoming an us-and-them situation, with me feeling more and more pushed out and somewhat bullied. I knew I was becoming paranoid, but I also knew that things felt 'off', and suddenly, I was very much on my own. I was being 'othered.'

By Christmas of 2007, I was beginning to feel very unhappy and lost. It was my first Christmas alone, and on Boxing Day, I was hit with a ton of grief as the reality of everything I had run away from came barreling back

and hit me square in the face. From being a valuable member of the team, suddenly I felt like an outcast and started hiding away in my hut rather than facing people (and drinking straight vodka from the bottle to numb the hideous emotions that flooded me). I remember one Sunday evening sitting and having a drink at the 'Lapa' bar with some of the paying guests (a writer and a doctor), as I couldn't face going back to the volunteer village. I felt depressed and couldn't stop crying and was almost hysterical, and the kindly American writer offered me a Valium. I had never taken Valium, but I am fairly sure it isn't ideal to have drunk a bottle of wine before taking it. But I did. There is very little I remember about the next few hours other than being reminded on the walkie-talkie that I was meant to be doing a baboon sleepover. I begged for someone else to do it instead, but the other co-ordinator was ice-cold and said no, so I staggered over to the main house to try and put nappies on the little baboons. I carried them to the newly commissioned sleepover room, which was empty other than a mattress on the floor. I realised I had been sick on my clothes, so stripped naked and huddled under the sleeping bag while the baboons ran riot around the room until they snuggled down with me. At some point, the door was flung open, the lights switched on, and someone was shouting at me. I wasn't sure if I was dreaming, but it was terrifying, as I was completely out

of it. The booze I knew how to manage, but combined with the drug, I was in virgin territory. The story goes that the temporary boss (who was in charge whilst the family were away for Christmas) had been told I was in an 'unfit state' and marched along to find out for herself. Bursting into the room, she found a naked woman passed out and two baby baboons leaping joyously around the room, smearing everywhere with shit, as my feeble attempts at nappy fixing had failed miserably.

Shame. Guilt. Shame. Guilt. Round and round we go.

In the space of two years, life had truly spiralled down from heaven to hell. I had started as the valuable volunteer and co-ordinator who could do no wrong, taking guests on tours when they had no guides available, creating a nativity play with the Bushmen's children (even though they spoke no English) and at one stage, being offered a full-time position at the centre. Now I sat in a "meeting to discuss my behaviour from the night before" with a circle of women who basically took turns to point out what I had done wrong. They did not mince their words. Some were gleeful, and others looked uncomfortable, but no one spoke up for me. I was hungover and had great chunks missing from the previous night, but in all honesty, I didn't feel I had done anything too horrendous. It had been Sunday night, and everyone else had the night off. It was the very first time

(in two years) that I had drunk alcohol and then had to take care of animals. Apart from their nappies falling off (and the shit on the walls!), nothing bad had happened. I did feel as though I had handed them something on a plate and provided a marvellous excuse to make an example of and get rid of me. The doctor was at the bar listening during this 'meeting' and even found my mobile number and called me at a later date to say it was a "Kangaroo Court" and absolutely appalling. If I had been sober, I would have argued my case and stood up for myself, but I felt agonisingly embarrassed, ashamed, and so alone. Looking back, yes, I did something very stupid, but the cruel and vindictive way it was dealt with left me feeling almost suicidal. I had no idea women could be so utterly cruel to other women and apparently enjoy it. Africa was no longer my refuge. I knew it was the end of this particular road (it was not made of yellow brick after all), and it was finally time to go home and face the music.

10

How low can you go?

When I left Namibia for the last time, I arrived back in drizzly London on 2nd January 2008. Rather than shiny New Year's Resolutions, I decided that, as my life was in tatters, I might as well really go full pelt into self-destruction mode. For a while, the drinking became even worse and the whole focus of my existence. It was astonishing to discover firsthand how a person can be so consumed with self-loathing that they give no care to their body whatsoever, and yet somehow, it continues to function. With hindsight, my drink pattern and response to it were pretty much the same each time: First glass of wine… ahhh, feeling a bit relaxed and definitely happier. Second drink; feeling even better mood-wise, with an extra boost of energy thrown into the mix. By drink 3, Shania Twain would be on, and there was a fair bit of

dancing around the house. If only I had managed to stop at that point, as it was always pretty downhill after that.

Drink 4 would often trigger some melancholy… out would come the laptop or phone so I could look at old photos of 'days of yore' when things were shiny and happy. Drink 5 was the time to make phone calls or texts… sometimes trying to sound upbeat and fun, but with an undercurrent of desperation and loneliness. The last glass in the bottle was the domain of self-loathing, recriminations, and disgust. On a good night, I would haul myself to bed without breaking anything. On a very bad night, I would be violently sick, wait for a while until my stomach felt better, and then start on the second bottle.

Lots of people drink a bottle of wine or two over a meal or with someone else, but these were on my own and often from start to finish in a couple of hours. I longed to be back working with animals, but there was not much call for lion rearing in Peckham Rye Park. I couldn't see any future for me, and the present was starting to close in and feel suffocating.

As time progressed, the ugly shadow side of my alcoholic 'gal pal' had really begun to show her true colours, and it was payback time with interest… hangovers, shaking, puking. The genie of the booze demanded a painfully high price for her work. She still permitted some emotional relief and dissociation from

my troubles, but I had to pay on a physical and practical level. Stomach and eye issues. Losing weight unhealthily, with most of my calories coming from alcohol. Too wobbly and paranoid to go out much in the daylight, in case people could see the horror of the 'Dorian Grey' portrait I was carrying around with me, taped to my back. Hanging out in late-night dives with all the others who came alive in the dark of the night, and falling asleep on buses heading to strange locations. Realising that I was drinking every day just to feel normal, and increasingly, having to drink more and more to reach that numb relief before crashing back into the sober waking hours filled with self-loathing and shame. Panicking about the gaps in my memory. Having no money and credit cards maxed out from buying emergency booze from the late-night corner shop. Of course, there is plenty more to the story… the numerous times I tried to 'just have one' and then woke up passed out on the sofa after two bottles of wine. The times I had a small drink while getting ready to go to a party, and then never got there, as I was too drunk to leave the house.

Panic. Guilt. Shame. Drink. Repeat.

Round and round we go, unable to get off the merry-go-round for fear of falling too far and not being able to get up again.

By this stage, I had stopped seeing friends and speaking to people at all, apart from hideous 'drunk dialling', which was filled with desperate emotion and followed by agonising embarrassment and shame (when I could actually remember having done it). No one wants to be friends with an out-of-control 41-year-old who is behaving like a wild teenager and refuses to listen to words of wisdom, no matter how lovingly given. I had nothing to offer anyone, and my world became smaller and smaller as I hid in my sordid house of booze, the thick red velvet curtains drawn 24 hours a day, and the rooms lit by candles as the light bulbs hurt my eyes. My doctor was aware of the situation but was unable to put me on the list for counselling until I had actually stopped drinking, and I couldn't. I had no money for private therapy. I had no money for anything except cheese, crackers, and wine. Even at my lowest ebb, I managed to get quality cheese and decent wine… clearly, I had some standards! I scoured websites of residential rehabs in the early hours, silently begging to miraculously be taken to one, as I knew I didn't have the strength to save myself.

I had willingly dug my own hole, and now, I was firmly stuck in it.

(Interval)

ACT 2

AFTER

11

Light at The End of The Tunnel

On that fateful, life-changing evening of 13th February 2008, I had been at a party in a pub. I had decided the week before to really try and get myself together and had taken on a job as a dog walker locally (the leaving 'do' was for the guy whom I was replacing). I had been shadowing him all week, walking in the woods with his five regular dogs. The walking, the dogs, and the trees were all starting to weave their healing magic, although I didn't realise it yet. As always, I drank like a sailor at the party and ate nothing (trying not to have too many extra calories!). The next thing I remember is waking up in the hospital. I had slipped in the ladies' room and sliced the back of my head open on a basin and was found a while later, lying unconscious in

a pool of blood. When the doctor was sewing up my head, I remember asking him, "Am I ok?" over and over. He looked at me sadly, and I was panicking that I was dying (ridiculous, as I was sitting up in a chair at the time). I obviously was ok in the end and got sent home in a cab with nine stitches in my head and an Olympic-sized headache. Alcohol had got me into this predicament, and unbelievably, the first thing I did when I got home was turn to alcohol to get me out of it. The following morning, after my 'day of reckoning' (and finally stone-cold sober), I had to drive a van for the first time, collect five big dogs, and then walk them around a beautiful woodland. I could hardly hold my head up with the pain, but I had never not shown up for work because of drinking, and I wasn't about to start then. This pattern of walking in nature with the dogs continued for 5 days a week for the next 6 months. Staying sober on weekdays was easy… I was driving and walking in the fresh air, and was shattered at the end of the day. Being amongst the trees made me feel dizzy and strange, but slowly my energy came back. The wood felt magical, and I could see a small ray of hope in the distance. I just went to bed very, very early before temptation could grab me. Weekends were harder. I fantasised about a glass of wine all the time and missed the patterns and habits of my previous life. I had to carve out new ones, which seemed dull. The days and evenings seemed very long and lonely

when I was sober all the time. There was too much time to think, and all my buried emotions began to pop up one by one, demanding attention, like an exhausting game of 'whack-a-mole'. When I was four months into sobriety, my go-getting Sagittarius sun personality came out of retirement and was tentatively in the driving seat. I was sober, vaguely healthy, and could see past the next few hours. Walking dogs had been a life-saving job for me, but I was cautiously starting to feel more optimistic. Maybe I could actually start my own dog business? I needed something I could do from home (that wasn't too taxing for my remaining undamaged brain cells), and dog grooming just about fitted the bill. I checked out the training options and was horror-stricken at the thought of wielding my scissors in a classroom with a bunch of 18-year-olds. Luckily, my hands no longer shook, but I knew I needed a calm environment where I wouldn't feel like some old dear who had wandered in off the street.

I discovered a British lady who had moved to Spain and set up a grooming salon there, where she offered bespoke training to 'mature' students. Come September, I was on another plane, this time to Malaga and onwards to a tiny village in Andalucia, where I then spent 4 weeks learning all the basics of grooming and practising on real-life dogs in the salon. I was pretty dreadful at the start, but felt proud of myself, living in a tiny apartment overlooking the sea and eating at tapas bars where every

night I had to turn away the glasses of wine they so eagerly plopped in front of me. I had no trees to offer me strength, so I fulfilled my nature healing sessions by taking long walks on the deserted beaches and sometimes shouting into the sea like a crazy lady. There wasn't much variety to the grooming requests… it was blazing hot, so all the owners just wanted their pets clipped short. By the end of the training, I was super-duper with clippers, but fancy styles were beyond me. I found Spain was a funny sort of dog place, very unlike the UK, in that they kept their pets in tiny apartments and did not seem to like them to be outside much. Every piece of grass I saw had a sign saying "Perros No". I think if I were a Perro, I would be saying no to living there, too.

Back in London, my new grooming business took off at a rate of knots, and after a second visit to sunny Spain for "advanced training", I was soon knocking out fancy-pants styles on breeds large and small. I was one of the first in my area to use organic pet shampoos, which were still so new in the UK at the time that I had to import them from Australia and the US. I wasn't keen on some of the traditional, rather insensitive methods of handling during grooming and decided to go 'off-piste' and become a holistic groomer. So began a 2-year part-time study period into canine behaviour with Sheila Harper and IPACS (International Programme for

Applied Canine Studies). This would lead to my second career, working for myself and rediscovering the joys of learning.

So… what had happened with the husband and family that disappeared for a while from my story? Well…. He was keeping a close eye on me from a distance throughout my fall and subsequent rise, and although he removed himself from the chaos, he ensured I had a roof over my head at all times. One of my brothers-in-law stayed available at the end of a phone during the dark days, but usually, I was too ashamed and embarrassed to call him. I wish I had found the courage to confide in him more, as he is an amazing therapist, but it was all a bit too close to home, and I really needed to talk to someone outside the family. The shame, guilt, sadness were overwhelming. I was perceived as the 'villain' of the piece and felt I needed someone neutral to hear my version. If only I had found a counsellor!

Christmas was fast approaching, and I was filled with another layer of terror. I was now 10 months sober and had never spent a Christmas without alcohol. My husband came and spent Christmas with me, and we ate proper food (which he cooked) as we glugged our way through a variety of pretty nasty non-alcoholic wines. Nowadays, there are some fabulous ones, but back in 2008, they were still fairly ropey. It was all strangely calm, and I was used to drama. A Christmas without fighting

over how many bottles of wine had been drunk. Was this how 'normal' people lived? We were treading on eggshells at the start, but my husband saw the changes were for real and basically never left again. We had somehow survived enormous tests and realised that we still wanted to be together.

By this stage, I felt I was a fairly okay person again, slowly rediscovering who I really was under the various facades I had adopted over the years. I thought sober me would be boring, but apparently, she is much nicer and more fun than crazy drunk me. Who knew?? I had managed to reframe my lifestyle and behaviours, but had not actually done any work on the deep emotions that had caused them in the first place. That was to be an ongoing process over many years.

Looking back, I don't know quite how I got through those first months alcohol-free, but it involved spending most of my time in the company of dogs and trees. There was true healing magic in that woodland. It was a place where I could think clearly, but for once, not be afraid of this clarity. Although I longed for my beloved baboons, it started to dawn on me that maybe I could make a future with animals in another way that was more practical, living in London. A plan was almost ready to hatch, but while it gestated, I had another problem to deal with.... My new 'addiction': ice cream!

12

Hunger

When I was drinking a lot of wine, I didn't have much of a sweet tooth. I hadn't realised how 'addicted' I was to sugar until I stopped the alcohol, and then my cravings were hideous and relentless: Gimme Booze, gimme biscuits, gimme booze, gimme cakes, gimme booze, gimme ice cream. As it turned out, ice cream was the victor, and I became utterly obsessed with Ben and Jerry's Half-Baked ice cream. It wasn't just a little bowl now and then; it was a whole tub, eaten slowly with a teaspoon, EVERY DAY. This happened at 4 pm daily and had become my new routine, something to look forward to as I counted the minutes of each long and painfully clear day of sobriety.

Hardly surprisingly, the pounds began to pile on, but I didn't notice for a while until none of my clothes fit and I had to start buying stuff with elasticated waists.

Even then, I turned a blind eye and just stopped looking in the mirror below my neck. How I loved to live in denial… first of my emotions, then of the harm I was doing to myself internally, and now, eating so unhealthily that I outwardly appeared as horrible as I felt inside. I was so exhausted all the time, as my body struggled with the daily dairy/sugar overload. Of course, I wasn't aware of this self-destructive strategy at the time; it was just something to look forward to in the endlessly stretching hours of the day before I could go to bed. I had discovered that eating ice cream numbed my brain and emotions in the same way that drinking did. Same plan, just different method of execution. I still couldn't face my pain. I just sugar-coated it.

Food and weight have been a recurring issue throughout my life since I was around 14 years old and started hitting puberty. I was already well into my training as an actress/singer/dancer, and particularly with the dancing side, there were no allowances made for puppy fat. I remember often coming home from school and having two "Limits" diet biscuits for my tea while doing my homework before heading out to dance classes. My mum did not enjoy cooking, and oven-ready food was still the fashion, so my meals were often 'Findus' pancakes and baked beans, so not particularly nourishing and extremely wind-causing! My mum had always been slim, possibly because she ate very little and

smoked a lot, so I didn't have the best role model for healthy eating.

Once I started theatre college as a full-time student, I was exercising so much that the weight stayed off reasonably well, but I remember nibbling Farley's Rusks to fill up a rumbling stomach and eating jars of baby's chocolate pudding, to have something sweet without too many calories. Even to this day, I eat desserts with a teaspoon to make them last longer. Nowadays, there is much more variety of shapes and sizes with dancers (although not so much in ballet), but when I was a student, you were expected to be thin, with big hair and lots of makeup at all times (well, it was the 80s!). No matter how hard I tried, I could never force my body to be the dancer I felt I was inside.... Legs too short, not enough 'turnout', and feet that did not have the right insteps. Boy, did I try to make myself fit the mould though... every evening at home, I would sit with my insteps wedged under the sofa, trying to get my feet to point more, and sleep in plastic trousers to try and lose weight off my hips and bottom. Tossing and turning at night in a cold, sweaty plastic was not conducive to restful sleep! Not good enough, not good enough, not good enough, the thoughts went round and round in my head. Be thinner, be funnier, be more.... *Something* and people will finally love you. I just didn't know what the 'something' was.

Although the training itself at my college was fantastic, we were impressionable and vulnerable teenagers, and nothing took away the terror of the public weighing sessions. I think they were designed to encourage us to stay out of the newly opened McDonald's across the road from the studio, but instead, they encouraged bingeing and starving. I was not naturally 'thin' but just about scraped by. Several eating disorders were born for others at this age, however, and although I developed a weird love/hate relationship with food, I never suffered the anorexia or bulimia of so many of my colleagues throughout my years as a performer. Instead, I yo-yo'd up and down with my weight, dieting to get roles and ballooning somewhat during the 'resting' times. I would sometimes struggle to eat in front of people, thinking they were judging me in some way, so preferred to hide away and enjoy food on my own. Definitely disordered eating, if not exactly an eating disorder. In my small world, thin always trumped healthy, no matter how you achieved it.

I feel sad looking back at my younger self when I see how desperately I tried to fit other people's ideas of how I should look. My self-esteem and self-confidence were totally dictated by the way other people saw me and whether they thought I was good enough. Even though, in reality, I was slim and pretty and talented, I usually looked in the mirror and decided that I was not good

enough, and this negative belief became a story that ingrained itself and seeped into every other area of my life. This was, of course, before social media, airbrushing, or even mobile phones, so the 24-hour pressure on young people to look or behave a certain way nowadays must be utterly unbearable at times. It was even then.

How I wish there had been more emphasis placed on how we are as people inside and on teaching us resilience, adaptability, and especially, self-worth, especially as girls and women. I had a single-parent mother who was intelligent but would play dumb to get people to do things for her. That strategy obviously worked for her (to some degree) but encouraged me to despise her fake neediness, which in turn, resulted in me refusing any help at all as I grew up, as I didn't want to appear weak and pathetic. Maybe this gave me some sort of inner strength or grit, but I did not have a female role model I could aspire to. Several amazing women did come into my life at different times, but for many years, I was so lost in my own feelings of inadequacy that I didn't learn the lessons they were offering.

13

Home

Apart from the amazing dog knowledge and understanding I acquired over the next couple of years, I also had another personal breakthrough. I often stayed on a farm when up in Staffordshire for the training, and when I opened my bedroom curtains every morning, I saw trees and sheep. It made me so calm and happy, and I could feel any stress melting away. Who knew that just looking at nature could have such a powerfully beneficial effect on my nervous system? One particular 4-day module was about reducing stress in dogs and was very illuminating in the way it related to humans, too. It was like a light bulb going off. I had no idea there was a different way of living where emotions could become balanced and harmonious. It sounded too good to be true, but I realised I wanted to find out for myself if it was possible.

My first morning back in London after the 'de-stress weekend', I opened my bedroom curtains and saw a car on fire and a group of guys whooping and hollering aggressively. A few weeks before that, I had witnessed a young man in the flats behind our garden beating his dog with a stick on a balcony and had got the RSPCA involved. I was then in fear that he would find out who had reported him and come and throw poison into my garden for our dogs (by now we had two fantastic Miniature Schnauzer puppies, Fred, 11 weeks old, and his sister, Lulu, came and joined the family at 6 months old). Maybe I was overly paranoid, but I realised that my stress levels were permanently high, and my adrenaline and cortisol never really had a chance to return to normal levels. I was starting to live in a permanent fight-or-flight state. I had started the canine behaviour training to help Lulu, as she was always "on" and unable to relax. I hadn't realised how similar we were and that helping her would lead to helping my wellbeing too.

I had loved being in London for many years, and it had been my safe place. It was paramount to live there when I was working in West End shows, but I now had a lot of very bad memories connected to our house, and I knew it was time for a change. I remembered back to when we had a Feng Shui expert come and give us advice on the energy in the house when we first moved in. This was in 1998, and despite emptying our bank accounts to

buy the house, I had insisted that we needed to have the energy cleansed by this very well-known expert, as I had a bad feeling in certain rooms. There had been a lot of violence and unhappiness in the house with the previous family, an aggressive divorce (forcing the sale of the house), and when we arrived, most of the bannisters were broken, and the front door was smashed in and held together with brown tape. F**K YOU was scratched into the woodwork. (You REALLY had to look beyond cosmetic appearances with this one!)

I explained to my husband that the Feng Shui specialist only charged £200 to come and do the magic stuff, and it would be worth it to start off our life there with a lovely clean slate. She looked around, checked directions with her compass, and we followed her around the house like a clapping centipede, clearing stuck energy in corners. She offered a few useful tips about hanging mirrors, red ribbons, and coins, but also said that all the doors needed to open in different ways on their hinges and that we should take an anticlockwise trip around the world before moving into the house (not so helpful). I was very keen on the principles of Feng Shui, though, and we were pleasantly surprised that she hung around to chat for ages afterwards, eventually staying for three and a half hours. It wasn't until the bill came that I realised she charged £200 an hour, and the £700 bill included plenty of chatting time!!

Maybe it was a forewarning of the problems that lay ahead, which would culminate in me being there alone, penniless, and at rock bottom, just like the previous lady owner. I had been trying to help her find a flat to move to, as she hadn't wanted to leave the house, but her husband had insisted on selling and getting his share. We had been in contact a fair bit during the sale process, and she seemed utterly broken and sad. She handed us the key on moving day and calmly said she was going off to kill herself (although she didn't, as we saw her locally many more times over the next few months). We were so excited to have our first house together, we didn't have a vast amount of patience with this poor, depressed lady, but it was certainly not the 'auspicious' moving-in day we had been hoping for with all our Feng Shui research and preparation.

There were definite strange vibrations in certain places in the house, and they remained so strong that after the first two nights, we never slept in the main bedroom again. Not that I am blaming my own spiral into darkness on the house itself, but I am fairly sure the energy in the space was not conducive to a happy life, with or without red ribbons and shiny coins.

The first 6 months were fun, though: stripping back to the bare bones of the house and discovering beautiful Victorian features, peeling off layers of vile Anaglypta wallpaper at midnight, and polishing old tiles around the

fireplaces. Having friends around for painting parties and murder mystery events. It was like an extended montage from a romcom, including us wearing cute 90s dungarees. Each 'scene' ended with us collapsing laughing on the sofa and, of course, drinking wine. Fifteen years later, there was less laughing, but I was finally coming out of the end of a very dark tunnel and blinking like a mole in the long-forgotten sunlight. Each carefully painted or papered wall had messy fingerprints from when I had staggered and tried to stop myself from falling. Glass-framed posters on the walls were cracked from when I fell down the stairs and knocked them all off mid-journey. The walls seemed to echo with howls of despair and endless nights of sobbing, no longer ringing with the music and laughter from nights of wild parties.

Somehow, the more I stepped back into the light, the less safe I felt in the house. I worried that it might swallow me back up and refuse to let me leave again. One day, after returning from the fresh air and sheep of Staffordshire, I looked at my husband and said, "Shall we move to the country?" and in the blink of an eye he said, "Ok".

And just like that, the decision that would shape the next stage of our lives was made.

14

Cover Me in Sunshine

That decision to up sticks and move to 'the country' was decided upon in March 2013; by September, we were there. Some of our family lived in Bath, so we drew a ring around it on a map and tootled up and down the motorway at weekends, looking at places within a 15-mile radius of the city. Somehow, having a new plan in a new place made me feel there was still something to look forward to. That maybe there was some new fun to be had. I just had to get away from all the people and places that reminded me of my darkest days. I never again went to the corner shop by our house. I just knew that the owner would silently hand me two bottles of wine in a blue carrier bag and thrust the credit card machine at me.

Our first new home was a little detached cottage in a beautiful Somerset village. It had a tiny wraparound garden and was surrounded by fields. "Great," we thought, "we can just walk the dogs there in all these lovely open spaces". Typical townies, we hadn't realised that much of the year, the fields would be filled with cows, peering over our little stone wall and mooing at the dogs (who were terrified of these giant gentle beasts). For a while, our city Schnauzers struggled with the vast space and the sound of horses clipping up and down the lane. Cars, motorbikes and lorries were fine, but strange animal noises, not so much. They eventually came to be very fond of the cows, though, sadly, they had a particular penchant for wolfing down steaming cow pats.

During this time, I was finding my feet and getting used to wellies. The West Country could well be renamed the Wet Country! I had left all my doggy clients in London and needed to start again from scratch, but it didn't take long to realise that not only was life in the country at a slower pace, but so was trying to build up a new business. Rather than being welcomed with homemade quiches and the like, "Blow-ins" from London were generally regarded with great suspicion and mainly avoided. It took quite a while for the locals to realise we were actually there to stay and not snooty weekenders.

I continued my canine behaviour training at a steady pace and also volunteered with local animal rescues. We had really wanted a Labrador to add to our family and somehow ended up with a beautiful 8-week-old puppy (Molly) and a 5-year-old rescue Labrador (Chewie) in the same week. For a while, I was wrapped up in the joy of living and working with animals, but a little part of me knew this wasn't quite the home I really wanted…. I always felt that I was on some kind of weekend away or mini break. After a very opportune series of events, we ended up viewing a house just a mile down the road, set on 3.9 acres of land. It had been on and off the market for a while, and by the time we walked around the land, we knew it was for us. The house needed a lot of work, but we went for it, and by February 2015, we were living in our dream place.

Over the next couple of years, we toiled and got plenty of blisters on our immaculate city hands. We planted trees and fixed endless fences (well, a nice man did, really) before welcoming three pygmy goats to the family (Vinnie, Leo, and Pablo). We had considered Alpacas instead, but I spent a day on a local Alpaca farm, and frankly, there was a lot of aggressive teeth action and spitting involved, plus they were a bit tall and terrifying (given that I am quite a short arse at 5ft 4"). It had been

a very busy few years with plenty of hard graft, so we decided to take a break from living like Tom and Barbara in "The Good Life" and try something very new.

15

Fun

On my 50th birthday morning, we woke up in a log cabin at the top of Finland, not far from the Russian border. We had broken our usual pattern of choosing the sunniest holidays we could find and decided to brave the freezing cold in order to see the Northern Lights (Little did we know that we could have hung on a few years and seen them for free in our back garden!) Sitting in bed wearing three layers, my husband handed me a little package, and I gently opened the paper with quite high expectations… well, it was my 50th after all!

Inside was a little plastic toy sheep.

I thought it must be a joke, and then the light bulb slowly flickered on in my chilled brain. It turned out that he had bought me three more pygmy goats (My nephews only had sheep in their toy farm, so he hadn't been able

to locate a representative plastic goat in time). It wasn't quite a Mulberry handbag, but it was the best gift I've ever had. I felt our original three wethers (neutered males) were rattling around in their paddock, and now we would have a proper 'flock.' It was to be a few months before the ladies joined us (Blossom, Berry, and Bramble), but in the meantime, we had a couple of days of adventure planned, including snowshoeing across the Lapish countryside, husky sledding, and a visit to a reindeer farm. All sounded marvellous, but during this once-in-a-lifetime trip, I discovered I was rubbish at quite a few things that should have been fairly straightforward, especially when doing them stone-cold sober!

Activity 1: Snowshoeing: Who knew that walking in snow was SO bloody difficult? After we had put on our four layers of outside gear, I really did look like a Teletubby. I would have said "Weeble", but they are not meant to fall down, and I did. Oh, so many times. This was supposed to be an easy activity, suitable for the 'over 50s', but snowshoes are evil things, like clown shoes on acid. They trick you with their apparent simplicity, and then the second you are not looking, they pull a fast one and wrap around one another. Everyone else in our group was sliding along satisfactorily and oohing and ahh-ing at the beautiful scenery, but every few steps, I would totter like a drunken sailor and then face-plant in

the snow. I had been a dancer, for heaven's sake… where was my balance and grace? Eventually, I had to take them off and then trudge along, up to my knees in the snow, carrying the blasted things. This was not a 'fun activity' as described, and my leg muscles were screaming.

Activity one

Snow: 1 - Michele: zero.

Activity two:

Husky Sledding**:** This was probably the part of the trip I was looking forward to the most. I imagined a romantic sleigh ride through the snow, with rosy cheeks and glowing eyes (like something out of Dr Zhivago but with dogs instead of horses). The huskies themselves were stunning beasts brimming with vibrancy and energy (too much energy, as it transpired), and the 'sleigh' was a piece of metal, where one person sat on the front, clinging on for dear life, and the other stood at the back, clinging on for dear life. The six sleds were one behind the other like a metallic caterpillar, and the instructor was very clear with his instructions.

"Don't let go, and don't fall off."

I opted for the sitting part first, as it seemed the easiest way to get the hang of it (and had a blanket), and with my husband being 6ft 2", he had the best hope of

slowing down proceedings with his foot, as apparently, that was somehow the way the brake worked. The huskies took off at a rate of knots, and we soon realised two things: the dog team in front was very slow, and our own team wanted to go very fast. I could hear a lot of huffing and cursing from behind, as my husband attempted to rein in our huskies, but it was impossible to turn round and see what was actually going on without an owl swivel head, plus my eyelashes were now encrusted with icicles. Exhilarating? Yes. Fun? Sort of. Freezing? I should coco!

Eventually, we all pulled into some sort of snowy lay-by to swap over. My husband gratefully sank into the seat with a sickly rictus grin on his face, and I stepped up the back, utterly convinced that driving a husky sled was somehow in my blood and second nature to me (why, I have no idea). Whatever is running through my veins is clearly not that kind of blood at all, as it very quickly turned icy cold and paralysing. Rather than enjoying the stunning scenery, I was gripping as hard as I could and reverting back to my Catholic childhood, monologuing 'Hail Marys' back-to-back, possibly with a bit of "It's a Long Way to Tipperary" thrown in for good measure. It was bloody terrifying!

As the slow-coach team in front started flagging even more, my huskies must have had a sneaky shot of something. They seemed to look at each other, and I am

sure I saw one of them wink as we reached the final straight, and they suddenly raced into 5th gear, with their ears and tongues lolling like astronauts encountering g-force. "Agghhhhh", I gurgled into the wind, forgetting all the instructions about where to put my feet to slow things down. As we sped round the corner, the sleigh went up on a bank, tipping us sideways. My feet slipped off the standing board, and I found myself being dragged along on my stomach, still holding onto the bar. I had failed miserably at the not falling off bit, but I was damned if I was going to let go too. After a few seconds of grazing the entire front of my body (and having my arms nearly yanked out of their sockets), I revised my plan and finally let go, lying spread-eagled on the ground screaming, "I'm off, I'm off." To my horror, I heard the rumbling of hooves (paws) behind me and voices shouting, "Get out of the way!" Like a true Hollywood stunt person, I rolled for my life as the next team of 6 huskies and their sled tore past, with the passengers rubbernecking like billy-oh.

When I finally uncovered my eyes and staggered to my feet, I could faintly make out the husky line disappearing into the distance like a Harry Potter train into the mist. I was left on the snowy platform and had no option but to start trudging in the same direction. On reflection, there was an awful lot of trudging on this trip. I rounded a corner after five minutes or so and was

greeted by a deathly white husband and an even paler guide, who clearly thought he had lost a client in a way that would not be useful in promoting the business; "come to Lapland for your 50th and get trampled to death by huskies"

I must say, I now truly appreciate the point of a sauna, as I spent a vast part of that evening in one, trying to bring life to my frozen everything. The following morning at breakfast in the lodge, tales of my exploits were tossed about in many languages with much jollity as I nodded and smiled through gritted teeth and attempted to bend my legs enough to sit down. There wasn't a vast amount of entertainment at the snow village, and clearly, for this weekend, I was it.

Activity Three

Reindeer Farm Visit**:** I bet you can hardly wait to discover the humiliating way I made an idiot of myself on this one! Well, dear reader, this time I did ok (one out of three ain't bad!). Except I couldn't eat the lunch as it was meat and couldn't drink the refreshments cos it had alcohol in it and couldn't do the lassoing cos I can't throw. Actually, it is extremely difficult to lasso a reindeer (or even a stick on a tree), so have a go before you judge! What I did do successfully, though, was have a very deep conversation with the Sami reindeer herder (mainly through mime and gurning), which resulted in

him lithely gadding over to a group of male deer (no trudging here) and picking up a freshly dropped antler. This was such a beautiful gift, I was moved to tears. It still sits on the mantlepiece in the dining room, covered in holly and berries to honour the lovely stag who timed his droppings so well.

Activity Four

Northern Lights: Um, well, we didn't actually see any as it was too cloudy. I would love to go back sometime and try again, if it wasn't for the very, very cold snow and the clown shoes and the incessant trudging. Hmm. Maybe I will stick with the sunny locations next time… after all, I'm fairly sure I know how to walk in flip-flops (although most holidays I have tripped over and twisted an ankle at least once, and in Crete last year I fell off a bus). Frank Spencer, eat your heart out! Some people really enjoy activities in the snow. I guess I am just not one of them. I will find my sober fun elsewhere.

16

Shores of Avalon

Back on grassy ground in Somerset, I had been helping dogs and owners for a while now (with holistic grooming, puppy classes, and canine behaviour issues), but I was aware of a yearning for something else. I was feeling stable in my life once again and decided I was ready to do some proper healing on myself. As a starting point, I signed up for a short crystal healing training with Earthworks School of Healing Arts (In Bradford on Avon) called "Follow the Rainbow". I had always loved crystals, but usually just collected ones I was drawn to and intuitively held them when needed or had them dotted about the house. That brief training opened a whole new world to me as I started to learn about 'vibrational healing,' colour therapy, and chakras. It was an excellent introduction, and I was hooked pretty quickly. In 2016, I discovered Touchstones School of

Crystal Healing and started a foundation-level crystal therapy practitioner training, which was held in person at the Chalice Well Gardens in Glastonbury (Somerset, UK). This was just the beginning of my connection with this magical town, known as the 'heart chakra of the earth,' and it was here that I would train as a 'Sacred Celebrant,' a gong practitioner, and a sacred oil practitioner. When I signed up for the 5-day foundation-level crystal training, I really saw it as a wonderful holiday pretending to be a course. Each day, I would get to spend my time in the Chalice Well Gardens and learn fascinating stuff whilst playing with beautiful crystals (I already had a few, but my collection was limited). Lauren D'Silva was the tutor, and I had read one of her books already (which was a little bit woo-woo for me at the time), so I expected a floaty, ethereal lady filled with waffle and wonder. In fact, I found an extremely grounded and no-nonsense teacher who happened to be an expert on crystals. The training blew my mind with its combination of geology, practical application, and seemingly magical healing. I did feel a bit of a fraud when everyone else declared they could see each other's auras. No matter how hard I squinted, I could see nothing and ended up slightly cross-eyed with a banging headache. However, it took me years to be able to do those 'Magic Eye'. Pictures, so I was determined to persevere. Crystal therapy was my first venture into holistic healing for

myself, and my curiosity and passion were certainly aroused. On the cautionary side, I discovered that crystal collecting is also very addictive (sigh).

I connected so strongly, not only with crystal therapy but with Lauren herself, and over the next couple of years, Lauren taught the Certificate and Diploma levels of the training at my home, both in the barn, and on the land. I was still absorbing everything for my own learning and, at that stage, had no intention of actually doing the homework and case studies to become a practitioner. Somehow, Lauren gently pushed me just enough so I could envisage being able to help other people, too. I reluctantly ploughed through the homework, and then suddenly found that with the case studies, I was enjoying it. "Maybe you do have it in you to help other people somehow?" a tiny, hopeful voice whispered in my head. "IMPOSTER!" another triumphant voice shouted. The shouty voice had the upper hand for the time being.

In 2020, the world turned upside down with the pandemic, and there were chunks of time when I could not work (I was still doing dog grooming and behaviour at this point and quietly studying crystals when 'shouty voice' was asleep). I had been supporting our dog 'Chewie' through a period of illness, which had resulted in seizures and the removal of an eye. As part of his care, I started using Bach Flower Essences to help him adjust

to the changes in his life. This was my first experience with vibrational essences, and in the same way that specific essential oils had helped him with his terror of fireworks and thunderstorms, these little bottles seemed to really help him relax. His last few weeks were very happy, and I was inspired to look further into training as an essence practitioner. My research led me to a woman named Sara Estelle Turner and her 'Essentially Flowers' vibrational essence practitioner diploma (now The School of Gaia for Healing) For the first time, the training was taken totally online and so began a 2-year adventure as I embarked on a transformational journey through my own life using a different vibrational healing modality. By summer 2022, I had graduated as an advanced practitioner and felt stronger, more confident and balanced. I had another tribe, wonderful women, all treading a healing path alongside me. I was truly ready to support others with their transformational healing experiences. The tiny hopeful voice was back in charge (and not so tiny anymore!)

I remember the first time I attended a 'gong and sound bath'. For anyone not familiar with this, basically, you sit on a chair or lie down on a mat, and the practitioner plays a variety of healing instruments with different vibrations. These are designed to take the participants to a state of physical, mental, and emotional relaxation. It is an ancient form of healing, known since

at least ancient Egyptian times. My first experience was not great. I had dragged my slightly unwilling husband along to a beautiful tithe barn, armed with yoga mats and a couple of fluffy blankets. The floor was wooden and harder than a rock, and the mat was very flimsy. We lay down expectantly, and within 5 minutes, my back had started to go into spasm. I started rolling around under my blanket, groaning as silently as I could. The barn doors were open to allow lurking COVID germs to escape, and a dog was barking incessantly. Sounds from the gongs and other instruments were amazing, but all I wanted to do was crawl towards the nearest exit and attempt to get off all fours. It was one of the longest hours of my life and quite clearly did not have the desired relaxing effect.

At the end of the slow torture, I turned to my husband, who was lying motionless in a state of bliss. "That was amazing," he mumbled, floating out of the building and towards the car. I hobbled furiously behind, dragging my blanket across the gravel. This was meant to be my 'thing'; how dare he find it fantastic, and I hate it. I was determined not to be beaten by a wooden floor. Sound baths were meant to be relaxing, and I WOULD bloody relax next time, one way or the other. After a few online visits to Amazon, we rocked up the following month, staggering under the weight of two rolled-up futons, blankets, pillows, and eye masks. And this time,

it *was* bliss. Once my brain stopped trying to control the sounds I was hearing and the thoughts they provoked, it threw its little brain hands in the air in resignation, and off I went into the wonderful world of the gong.

As someone who has struggled with some other types of meditation (the calmer I try to be, the faster my mind spins), I was fascinated to find that sound healing bypasses our busy 'monkey minds' and, like it or not, gently eases us out of our day-to-day cortisol-spiked existence and into a more harmonious state of balance. Sometimes, I felt that I was welded to the ground, and on other occasions, I floated away, meeting random people in visualisations or seeing beautiful colours. Each session was different, but more and more, my sleep became filled with fabulously lucid dreams, and I generally felt a calmer, happier person.

This was what I wanted to be able to do for other people. To me, sound healing was the ultimate tool for transformation.... As fast as drugs or alcohol to change how you feel, but with no comedown or hangover. Playing is intuitive and unprescribed once you have learned some skills with the instruments. And so, this was the birth of my newest venture and the start of my training in a variety of instruments, including crystal bowls, shamanic drum, Tibetan bowls, voice, and gong. I loved using them all, but my absolute passion was the gong (It would be the most expensive instrument,

naturally!) Of course, I could justify my newfound gong addiction as it was my work! It was healing and good for me, and clearly, it was a vocation. Yes, I really did need four gongs! (now five!!)

With my various trainings completed and my new, fledgling holistic business gradually forming, I now had my four pillars of wellbeing in place: Crystals, essential oils, vibrational essences, and sound therapy, all creating a safe structure around my nature 'healing temple'. These had all helped me find my way in my new life. Now, it is time to put my money where my mouth is and see if I can actually make a difference for others in the big, wide world. The new adventure begins…

Egypt (2025)

As I breathe in deeply, the sticky air assaults my nostrils with the atmospheric whiff of spicy food, incense, and camel poo. I feel happy and whole, as though I have returned to my spiritual home. Ahead of me, the pyramid of Menkaure is shimmering like a mirage in the desert, calmly welcoming me as I stagger down the steep steps to its heated heart, ready to create my vibrational essence. Once the alchemy is complete, I climb back into the present, blinking in the sunlight and clutching my glass bottle of water concealed in its oilskin bag. I keep walking through the desert, trying not to be distracted by the hypnotic presence of the Sphinx,

offering her riddles and taking no prisoners. It has been almost 30 years since I first came here with my husband on our honeymoon when we rode skinny-but-lively horses around the pyramids (we were pretty lively ourselves at the time, if not that skinny). We camel-trekked through the desert with scarves artfully wound around our bonces and glided down the Nile Agatha Christie-style, our spirits gorging on the endless wonder and magic of Egypt. This time, I am in a bigger body, and my clothes stick to me uncomfortably as the sweat slowly trickles into every orifice. Not pleasant. The osteoarthritis in my toes and hands is tingling aggressively in the warm January sun, and the pain from the fibromyalgia is scratching at every nerve end. I feel old and slow and couldn't hop on a camel again for love or money. And yet, I feel happy. I am glad to be still alive after the hairy, scary journey I took myself on since my previous visit to Cairo. This morning, I caught sight of someone in the window of one of the ubiquitous perfume shops, and my heart sank a little when I remembered that this rather dumpy middle-aged woman staring back at me was me. I still get surprised. Inside, I don't feel the way I look. I feel young, beautiful, and free, as though I could turn cartwheels in the dust. I am aware of every thought and emotion with cut-glass clarity. Sometimes, these are as painful as my body, and I yearn for a temporary reprieve. But then I remember the

alternatives and know this is a price I will gladly pay to be back in Egypt once again. Happy, sober, and definitely worthy of love.

We sit on the small balcony, staring out into the desert and eating Koshari with plastic spoons. It is the most delicious meal I can remember having. There is a sultry breeze, and the street below is a cacophony of noise… the weary grumbles of camels and horses after their long day ferrying tourists around the Sahara. Lights begin flashing, and I hear a booming theatrical voice declaring, "You have come tonight to the most fabulous and celebrated place in the world!". It is the famous 'Sound and Light Show' of Giza. Grandiose and ridiculously camp, but totally right for the dramatic backdrop of the pyramids. The breeze picks up, and I turn to the Brown-Eyed Man beside me, Dan. He holds my hand and smiles.

I hear a whisper, maybe from the Sphinx herself:

"You are worthy of love".

You are ENOUGH.

ACT 3

NOW

17

Reflection

If you have stayed with me to this point, I thank you and congratulate you on your grit while remaining on this uncomfortable ride. If you have reached a very low point or even completely lost everything in your life (including your self-respect), my heart is with you. If any kind of addiction or self-sabotage has been part of your experience, then maybe you will have been able to relate in some way to this tale. Some of you will understand how it is to live your life not feeling 'good enough'.

So, my husband had a read of the first draft of this book and offered plenty of 'constructive criticism'. He is very good with words and an avid reader, so much of it was invaluable. Then he paused and put his serious face on. "But what is the point of the book? He said. Why did you write it?" I felt a bit ruffled. "Well, surely the book is self-explanatory?" I said. He paused and

searched for the right words so as not to offend my fledgling author's vulnerability. "Um, well, it is just like a long letter or journal. I can see why it was cathartic to get it all out, but why would anyone else want to read it?"

He had a point. I guess I wrote this book for several reasons.

- To actually put the pain of my transformation down in black and white and own it.
- To recognise my achievement
- To honour the people who helped me along the way
- To have the courage to stand up and show myself with no filters, masks, or excuses
- In the hope that it may inspire, encourage, or touch even just one other person in the world

Looking back at the darkest days, I often wonder how I could have dealt with it differently and taken a less painful route. I would absolutely NOT recommend doing what I did and stopping alcohol 'cold turkey' style. So much more support and help is available nowadays, so do ask for it if you find yourself in the same position. I really struggled physically those first few weeks and hadn't realised how dangerous it could have been. In my case, I was lucky, but there are other ways to be kinder and gentler with your recovery. The only times I called

an AA line were when I was drunk and tearful and

basically just needed someone to talk /cry/vent at. Maybe I would have really benefited from attending a few meetings in the early days, and maybe I will go along to one in the future. A good friend of mine stopped drinking quite a few years after me, when his life had also fallen apart. He found AA incredibly helpful, and now, he sponsors other people. Horses for courses, I guess.

For me, this book is like coming out of a cave where I have been hiding, reflecting, and transforming for about 17 years (too long for the caterpillar into butterfly comparison?) I have been holding onto a heavy load for most of my life, like an Oak tree supporting hundreds of other species. Over time, I have gradually been lightening it and letting go of all the painful broken pieces. It has been very hard to let go (after all, I am the daughter of a hoarder), and to do that, supportive new strong branches have needed to grow, which has taken time.

There are still more layers to uncover, some so deep that they are not quite ready to face the cold light of day. There may well be a second book simmering in the pot, but for now, I feel quite naked enough with all the honest sharing and baring. I hope you, the reader, will be kind, as my soft underbelly is very exposed at present!

So, what, you may ask, am I doing now with all my experience and the new life path it offered me? Well, I still spend most of my time in the company of dogs and trees on our small 'wellbeing retreat' in Somerset. We also have pygmy goats, chickens, and over the years, a motley crew of rescued cats. I have a 'healing yurt', where I offer gong and sound baths, either 1-2-1 or in small groups. I have learned to work with the energy of the moon cycles, the seasons, and astrology. At the Spring Equinox in 2023, after 9 months of beautiful self-discovery with a group of heart-centred women, I 'emerged' as a modern-day 'Priestess of the New Earth'. A long way from sleeping drunk in a shop doorway because I couldn't remember where I lived.

The more I work with women, the more I understand that there are so many deep emotional traumas that we hold deeply buried, often smouldering away beneath a fragile veneer of 'I'm okays' and desperately gulped glasses of wine. Sometimes, just having someone create a safe, non-judgmental space and listen to us is all that is needed to start the healing. We don't want someone to 'fix' us… We are not broken; we are just using coping mechanisms that have served us in the past but may have reached the end of their usefulness. A quiet place in nature, a gentle ear, and a warm heart can work wonders in this busy day and age. This is how Wild Oak Wellbeing came along. Nestled

beneath ancient oak trees, I have a room full of crystals and essences and a yurt full of love, feathers, sticks, stones, and gongs. One day, I hope to have a woodland to walk in alongside other women, so that they too feel the magic of nature as it reignites their hope and fills them with strength.

For so long, I felt that I had to juggle life on my own, as I lacked trust and feared being hurt. Once I could finally tune in to my heart, intuition, and higher self (with the help of nature), I could discern whom I could ask for help, guidance, and teaching. Invariably, these were people who had already been on their own healing journey, and they had great compassion, having reached a stage where they had something to pass on to others. I feel that I, too, have finally reached the stage to be there for other women who are struggling.

By the way, I haven't morphed into some kind of worthy saint! I still have the same weaknesses and cravings, but my main addictions nowadays are Earl Grey Tea and almond macarons. Yes, too much caffeine and sugar, but a vast improvement on what came before. My binges now are usually watching horror films or ones with Vikings. I enjoy my drama vicariously these days and get my adrenaline buzz from watching fictional sagas of other people going through their trials and tribulations and (sometimes) coming out the other end

in one piece. I prefer my own life to be calmer and more restful. Maybe it seems a bit less adventurous, but it makes me happy, and I feel I already had a lifetime's worth of drama and excitement; someone else's turn now.

The next chapter of my life is especially unexpected, as at the grand old age of 56, I have finally gone to university to study a degree in Integrative Counselling. I haven't done any academic work since my O-levels forty years ago, so this is an enormous challenge in every way. I am especially interested in the latest therapeutic developments for working with depression, eating disorders, and, of course, addictions, and I am currently researching the neuroscience of using sound and nature therapy to help with these issues.

I have my husband and his (**my**) lovely family supporting me in all my new 'adventures'. My life is filled with growth, learning, and peace.

My heartfelt wish is that this book will show that there is always hope for transformation, recovery, and a new, better way of living where you can feel good about yourself. Where you feel totally seen, understood, and loved despite everything that has gone before. Even from the winey dregs at the very bottom of a bottle, it is possible to crawl back out. Help is there if you want it (and if you are ready), and miracles and magic are still alive today. I know, from experience.

And you don't need a magic lamp. Or even sparkly red shoes (although they do help!)

I like myself and know I am just a work in progress, like everyone else.

Oh yes, dear reader. I am more than enough.

And so are you.

(Curtain)

About the Author

Michele is a holistic wellbeing practitioner and mindfulness teacher. She is currently pursuing a degree in integrative counselling. She offers retreats and healing transformational packages using sound therapy, vibrational essences, crystals, and essential oils. She has a yurt and treatment room beneath ancient oak trees in Somerset, UK.

She is now also an author (woohoo!).

When not studying, writing, or playing gongs, Michele can be found beneath a pile of animals, usually covered in mud and dog lick.

www.wildoakwellbeing.co.uk

Email: wildoakwellbeing@gmail.com

Story Soundtrack

There is a soundtrack to accompany this book, as each chapter title is also a song performed by an amazing woman. There is no particular theme, other than the lyrics connecting with something in the essence of the chapter and meaning something to me. Please feel free to listen to them before, after or while you are reading if you are so inclined. Much heartfelt gratitude to the wonderful artists who performed them and for the inspiration they brought me along the way.

1. Genie in a bottle (Christina Aguilera)
2. Dysfunctional Family Holidays (Lana Brown)
3. Windmills of Your Mind (Barbra Streisand)
4. No Business like Show Business (Ethel Merman)
5. Soulmate (Natasha Bedingfield)
6. Bigger than the Whole Sky (Taylor Swift)
7. Lions and Tigers and Bears (Booze!) oh my! (Wizard of Oz)
8. Last Chance (Emily Kinney)
9. Spinning Wheel (Shirley Bassey)
10. How low can you go? (LP)
11. Light at the End of the Tunnel (Kate Vogel)
12. Hunger (Florence and the Machine)
13. Home (Nichelle Lewis, Broadway cast of The Wiz)

14. Cover Me in Sunshine (Pink)
15. Fun (Little Sis Nora)
16. Shores of Avalon (Tina Malia)
17. Reflection (Christina Aguilera)